Clinical
Essentials of
Pain Management

Clinical Essentials of Pain Management

Robert J. Gatchel

American Psychological Association | Washington, DC

Published by
American Psychological Association
750 First Street, NE
Washington, DC 20002
www.apa.org

To order
APA Order Department
P.O. Box 92984
Washington, DC 20090-2984
Tel: (800) 374-2721
Direct: (202) 336-5510
Fax: (202) 336-5502
TDD/TTY: (202) 336-6123
Online: www.apa.org/books/
E-mail: order@apa.org

In the U.K., Europe, Africa, and the Middle East, copies may be ordered from
American Psychological Association
3 Henrietta Street
Covent Garden, London
WC2E 8LU England

Typeset in Goudy by World Composition Services, Inc., Sterling, VA

Printer: Book-Mart Press, Inc., North Bergen, NJ
Cover Designer: Naylor Design, Washington, DC
Technical/Production Editor: Rosemary Moulton

Library of Congress Cataloging-in-Publication Data

Gatchel, Robert J., 1947–
        Clinical essentials of pain management / Robert J. Gatchel.
           p. cm.
        Includes bibliographical references and index.
        ISBN 1-59147-153-2 (alk. paper)
        1. Pain—Treatment. I. Title.

  RB127.G38 2004
  616′.0472—dc22   2004013978

British Library Cataloguing-in-Publication Data
A CIP record is available from the British Library.

Printed in the United States of America
First Edition

To Margaret McDermott and Mary McDermott Cook, for their continued support of pain management and research at the Eugene McDermott Center for Pain Management, the University of Texas Southwestern Medical Center at Dallas, and their vision that no one in this world should hurt or needlessly suffer from pain.

CONTENTS

PREFACE

As discussed in this book, pain is one of the most prevalent symptoms reported in medical settings and is the most frequent reason for physician consultation. In fact, physicians are now required to consider pain as a "fifth vital sign" (added to pulse, blood pressure, core temperature, and respiration), which now must be officially documented in medical charts. Pain exacts an enormous economic cost and emotional toll on millions of Americans. Because of these factors, the U.S. Congress designated the years 2001–2010 as the "Decade of Pain Control and Research."

Fortunately, a number of important advances are now being made in the areas of etiology, assessment, treatment, and prevention of chronic pain. What has prompted these advances has been a major paradigm shift in medicine, spearheaded primarily by groundbreaking work in pain management. The shift has been away from the traditional, but overly simplistic, biomedical reductionistic approach to medical disorders to a more heuristic and comprehensive biopsychosocial perspective. This perspective, in contrast to the biomedical model's sole emphasis on disease, focuses on illness, which is the result of the complex interaction of biological, psychological, and social variables. This interaction shapes a patient's perceptions and response to illness and accounts for the diversity in illness expression across patients. This biopsychosocial perspective is the common thread throughout the fabric of this book.

With this important paradigm shift, there has been a recent explosion of clinical interest and documentation of the most effective approaches to the assessment and treatment of pain syndromes. Paradoxically, though, it has been difficult for many practitioners of pain management to keep abreast of the most current state of the art and evidence-based methods now available. The major purpose of this book is to provide such information, as well as the nuts and bolts of how to administer clinically effective methods of pain assessment and management. Indeed, this book is designed to provide practical clinical guidance to health care professionals who are working (or are considering working) in pain management settings.

The various chapters of this book have been written for practitioners who desire information about the most effective empirically documented methods of pain assessment and management that can be applied in the clinical arena. They will be of particular relevance and interest to health care professionals (physicians, dentists, nurses, psychologists and psychiatrists, physical therapists, chiropractors, occupational therapists, and case managers), whether they see only a small number of patients with pain or whether the majority of their practice is devoted to this population. The chapters provide practical clinical information and guidelines, ranging from the now widely embraced biopsychosocial conceptualization of pain to important assessment and treatment approaches as well as practical issues, such as reimbursement for pain management services. I have accumulated a wealth of clinical experience over the past 20 years working in diverse pain management settings, and I hope that my insights, combined with the empirically based information I present, will provide a pragmatic guide for health care professionals who are interested in clinical pain assessment and management.

Of course, no book of this type is possible without the aid of many dedicated people. I am especially grateful to a number of colleagues who contributed helpful clinical material and suggestions, especially Peter Polatin, Anna Wright, Martin Deschner, and Randy Neblett, as well as Lewis Calver, who contributed to the illustration artwork. I also thank the book reviewers for their thoughtful comments and suggestions. In addition, I appreciate the help and support I have received from the American Psychological Association's publication staff, particularly Susan Reynolds and Ed Meidenbauer. Finally, I greatly laud the outstanding work of Carol Gentry in helping to bring this book to fruition.

I

THE CONCEPTUAL
FOUNDATIONS OF
PAIN MANAGEMENT

1

HISTORICAL OVERVIEW

Pain is an even more terrible lord of mankind than even death itself.
—Albert Schweitzer, *On the Edge of the Primeval Forest* (1922)

Attempts to treat pain have a long history. As has been highlighted, the quest to understand and control pain has been a significant human pursuit since earliest recorded history (Gatchel, 1999). Today, pain is still a very pervasive medical problem and, as Gatchel and Turk (1996) noted, is associated with the following statistics: It accounts for over 80% of all physician visits; it affects more than 50 million Americans; each year, an estimated 176,850 patients seek treatment in pain centers in the United States alone; and there is a cost of over $100 billion annually in health care and lost productivity (including lost earnings, decreased productivity, and increased health care utilization expenses and disability benefits). Recent data also indicate that the number of Americans using pain management programs increased 64% from 1998 to 2000 (Marketdata Enterprises, 2001). Also, the number of patient visits to all types of pain programs increased 26% in 2000, with new patients accounting for 16% of the total gain. On the basis of interviews with more than 197,000 individuals assessed in the National Health Interview Survey, conducted in 1998, Pleis and Coles (1998) estimated that, in the 3-month period prior to the survey, 28% of the adult U.S. population had experienced pain in the lower back, 16% had experienced migraine or severe headaches, 15% had experienced pain in the neck region, and 4% had experienced pain in the face or jaw area. Moreover, overall, 32% of the sample reported limitations that affected their ability to walk a quarter of a mile, stand for 2 hours, reach over their heads, use their fingers to grasp small objects, or lift or carry 10-pound items. In addition, estimates indicate that more than 30 million to 50 million American adults experience chronic or acute recurrent pain (Joranson & Lietman, 1994). Finally, the total annual costs of chronic pain (including treatment, disability payments, legal fees, and lost work days) have been estimated to range from $150 billion to $215 billion in the United States (National Research Council, 2001; U.S. Bureau of the Census, 1996).

Besides these enormous costs to society, a great deal of emotional suffering is experienced by patients with pain. Thus, it is no wonder that there have been constant attempts to develop the most effective pain management techniques. There is now a mandate from the Joint Commission on the Accreditation of Healthcare Organizations (2000) requiring that physicians consider pain a *fifth vital sign* (in addition to pulse, blood pressure, core body temperature, and respiration). Pain severity must be documented using a pain scale; one that can easily be used is presented in Exhibit 1.1. In addition, the patients' own words describing their pain, pain location, duration, aggravating and alleviating factors, present pain management regimens and their effectiveness, effects of pain, and the patient's pain goal, as well as the physical examination, all must be documented during the initial assessment. As well, with proclamations from the nonprofit American Pain Foundation's "Pain Care Bill of Rights" (see Appendix 1.2; http://www.painfoundation. org), a new zeitgeist has emerged, calling for appropriate management of all types of pain, malignant and nonmalignant.

HISTORICAL OVERVIEW OF THE MIND–BODY RELATION

As I reviewed in an earlier book (Gatchel, 1999), the history of attempts at understanding the etiology and treatment of pain parallels the historical changes that have occurred in medicine in general. During the Renaissance period, with the great revolution in scientific knowledge in the areas of anatomy, biology, physiology, and physics, a biomedical reductionism perspective developed. This was primarily due to the new approach in the investigation of physical phenomena that emerged during this period. Projects based on the dissection of the human body and associated experimentation stimulated a revolution in a scientific method of gaining more knowledge through careful observation, experimentation, and objective quantification. This was an attempt to replace traditional approaches that relied merely on common sense, mythology, or outdated dogma. Various revolutionary works appeared at this point in time, such as *De Humani Corporis Fabrica*, a seminal anatomy textbook published in 1543 by the Dutch physician Andreas Vesalius. In 1628, English physician William Harvey discovered that blood circulates in the body and is propelled by the

EXHIBIT 1.1
Pain Assessment Questionnaire

I. Location and intensity of pain

1. Indicate all of the places that you feel pain

    Right   Left   Left   Right

_____

_____

_____

_____

_____

2. Which location has the most intense pain?

_____

3. What words best describe your pain? (Circle)
   a) mild/distracting   b) moderate/uncomfortable
   c) strong/upsetting   d) severe/unbearable

4. On a scale of 0 to 10, 0 = No pain, 10 = worst possible pain;

| 0 | 1 | 2 | 3 | 4 | 5 | 6 | 7 | 8 | 9 | 10 |

  no pain   worst pain possible

   What number best describes the way you feel *now?* _____
   The usual, *average* amount of pain? _____
   Pain at its worst? _____

5. What sensations best describe the type of pain you are feeling? (Circle)
   a) sharp or dull
   b) deep, aching, cramping sensation, throbbing
   c) hot or burning, tingling, prickling (like area has "fallen asleep"), piercing ("pins & needles"), stabbing

   Patient Name: _____ Date: _____

II. Timing of pain

6. When did you first notice pain?
   Month _____ Year _____

7. Was the onset of pain immediate, or did it gradually build up?

_____

8. Is your pain constant or does it come and go?

_____

9. If your pain isn't constant, how often does the pain occur?

_____

(continues)

EXHIBIT 1.1 *(Continued)*

III. Lifestyle factors

10. How much time do you spend thinking and talking about your pain?

_____ Hours/Day

11. Has the pain affected your lifestyle or limited your function in any way? Check all that are affected:

_____ Strength   _____ Mood

_____ Sleep   _____ Appetite

12. Does moving the affected body part make the pain worse?

_____ Yes   _____ No

Have you noticed any other aggravating factors?

_____

13. What ways have you found to relieve your pain (such as elevating the affected body part, applying hot or cold compresses, or taking a pain relieving medication)?

_____

14. Are you taking any treatments or medication for your pain? If so, list them here:

_____

_____

_____

Note. From Watson Pharmaceuticals, n.d. Copyright Watson Pharmaceuticals, Inc., 311 Bonnie Circle, Corona, CA 92880. Reprinted with permission.

heart. Such influential works highlighted the significant advances in the view that the body could be explained by mechanisms. This viewpoint stimulated what was then called the *biomedical reductionism* approach. Advocates of this approach argued that concepts such as the mind or soul were not needed to explain physical functioning or behavior. This approach also stimulated a great new revolution in knowledge, with sciences such as anatomy, biology, and physiology—all of which would be based on the principles of scientific investigation—evolving simultaneously.

This new mechanistic approach to the study of human anatomy and physiology began to foster a dualistic viewpoint that the body and mind function separately and independently. Before the Renaissance period, physicians had approached the understanding of mind–body interactions in a more holistic way. These physicians also served the multiple roles of philosopher, teacher, priest, and healer. One historical figure often viewed as popularizing and solidifying this dualistic viewpoint is the 17th-century French philosopher René Descartes (1596–1650), who postulated that the mind or soul was a completely separate entity parallel to, and incapable of affecting, physical matter or somatic processes in any significant or direct way. Such a dualistic viewpoint gained additional acceptance during the 19th century, with the discovery that microorganisms caused certain diseases. This novel and revolutionary biomedical reductionism philosophy of medicine then became viewed as the only acceptable basis for explaining diseases through an understanding of mechanical laws and physiological processes and principles.

Although the above reductionistic approach to medicine played a valuable role in bringing medicine out of the Dark Ages, so to speak, and prompting significant discoveries and maturation of the field as a science, it had a subsequent stifling effect on the field during the 19th and 20th centuries, with the advent of clinical research emphasizing the importance of taking into account mind (or psychological factors) for a more thorough understanding of a physical disorder. A discussion of the emergence of this *biopsychosocial* approach is presented later in this chapter.

EARLY THEORIES OF PAIN

Descartes initially conceptualized pain as a specific type of activity in the sensory nervous system. He viewed the pain system as a "straight-through" channel from the skin directly to the brain. In his analogy, a pain system was imagined to be like the bell-ringing mechanism in a church: If someone pulls the rope at the bottom of the tower, then the bell rings at the top. Thus, he proposed that, if a flame is applied to the hand, it sends particles in the hand into activity, and that motion is transmitted up the arm and neck into the head, where it activates something like an alarm system. The person feels the pain and responds to it. This purely deductive theory of pain physiology, even though it lacked any empirical evidence, influenced the study and management of pain for the next few centuries.

A much more formal model of this pain process, called the *specificity theory of pain*, was subsequently proposed by von Frey in 1894 (Gatchel, 1999). This theory proposed that sensory receptors were responsible for the transmission of specific sensations, such as pain, touch, warmth, and pressure, and that the various receptors had different structures that made them differentially sensitive to various types of stimulation. Therefore, pain was perceived as having a specific central, as well as peripheral, set of mechanisms—similar to those that operate for other bodily senses.

At about this same point in time, Goldscheider proposed an alternative model, which he called the *pattern theory of pain* (Gatchel, 1999). Goldscheider conceptualized pain sensations as being the result of transmissions of nerve impulse *patterns* that were produced and coded at the peripheral stimulation site and that the differences in the patterning and quantity of peripheral nerve fiber discharges produced differences in the quality of sensation. He assumed that the experience of pain was the result of the central nervous system's coding of nerve impulse patterns and not simply the result of a specific connection between pain receptors and pain sites.

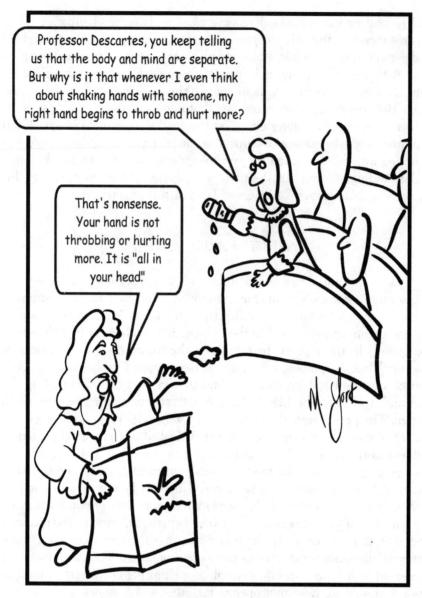

The outdated dualistic view of mind and body.

Although von Frey's and Goldschneider's theories were initially accepted by the scientific community, there was insufficient evidence accumulated over time to totally explain pain, even though there was some level of support for each theory (Gatchel & Weisberg, 2000). Moreover, various empirical findings could not be accounted for by either of these two theories. Again, this strict, mechanistic, biomedical reductionist approach to medicine began to subside somewhat because of the advent of important work implicating the role of psychosocial factors in medical disorders. Indeed, Bonica (1953) pointed out the various shortcomings of both of these earlier two purely mechanistic models of pain. As Loeser (2003, p. 5) succinctly stated: "The biomedical model is fatally flawed, as it does not consider events outside the patient as relevant to disease in general or pain in particular."

MORE RECENT THEORIES OF PAIN

During the last 30 years, there have been major advances in the understanding of the close interaction of physiological and psychosocial processes in pain perception. The transition of these advances, which is discussed next, is depicted in Figure 1.1. These advances started from the early biomedical reductionist theories of Descartes, von Frey, and Goldschneider to more useful models of pain that took into account the complementary interactions of biological and psychosocial factors.

The Gate-Control Theory of Pain

The first major theory of pain, called the *gate-control theory of pain*, emphasized the close interaction between psychosocial and physiological processes affecting pain and was proposed by Melzack and Wall (1965). The theory accounted for many diverse factors involved in pain perception. This model of pain describes how thoughts, feelings, and behavior affect pain. Pain is a subjective experience that varies across people and different situations. The pain message begins at the site of injury, then a signal of pain is transmitted to the brain, and then an individual becomes aware of the pain sensation.

A "gate" located in the brain determines a person's perception of pain. This gate can be opened or closed, and it determines the amount of pain one feels. Coping strategies can "close the gate," increase one's ability to cope, and give a person more control over his or her pain. Thoughts that "open the gate" are focusing on the pain, negative thinking, and nonconstructive thinking. Feelings that open the gate include stress, tension, sadness, hopelessness, helplessness, and anger. Many people experience these feelings at some point in time; this is a normal reaction when experiencing prolonged pain. But it is important to identify your negative, self-defeating thoughts and feelings to ensure that you do not stay focused on them.

Behaviors that can open the gate include poor nutrition, inactivity, inadequate sleep, smoking, and lack of exercise. These factors predispose a person to pain and increase one's vulnerability to pain and to more intense pain.

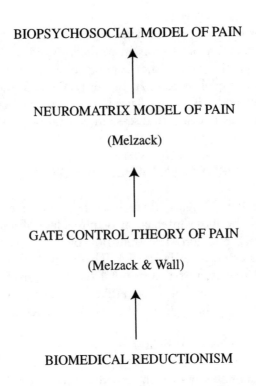

BIOPSYCHOSOCIAL MODEL OF PAIN

NEUROMATRIX MODEL OF PAIN

(Melzack)

GATE CONTROL THEORY OF PAIN

(Melzack & Wall)

BIOMEDICAL REDUCTIONISM

Goldschneider's *Pattern Theory of Pain*

Von Frey's *Specificity Theory of Pain*

Descartes' Mind–Body Dualistic Perspective and
Straight-Through Model of Pain

Figure 1.1. Summary of the advances in theories and models of pain, starting with biomedical reductionism models to the present biopsychosocial model of pain.

The primary contribution to the scientific community of the gate-control theory of pain was the introduction of the importance both of central nervous system and psychosocial variables in the pain perception process. It highlighted the potentially significant role of psychosocial factors in pain perception (Melzack, 1993). Although the physiological processes involved in the gate-control model were initially challenged, and suggestions were made that the model was incomplete (Nathan, 1976), additional research accumulated that prompted some revision and reformulation of the original model (Wall, 1989). Nevertheless, the gate-control model of pain has proven quite resilient in the face of recent scientific data and theoretical challenges, to the point that it still provides the most heuristic perspective of the wide range of pain phenomena encountered in medical settings today. Of course, like most scientific models, a more refined model will most likely evolve over time as the understanding of pain neurophysiology, neurotransmission, and opioid receptors increases. It often is clinically useful to review the gate-control theory of pain with patients so that they can develop a better understanding of some of the basic mechanisms of pain.

The Neuromatrix Model of Pain

Melzack (1999) extended the gate-control theory of pain and integrated it with models of stress (which Selye, 1950, first introduced). This *neuromatrix theory* assumes that pain is a multidimensional experience and is produced by specific patterns of nerve impulses generated by a widely distributed neural network, or *neuromatrix*. Nerve impulse patterns can be triggered either by peripheral sensory input or centrally, without peripheral stimulation. The final neuromatrix is determined and modified by multiple factors: genetic, sensory experiences, and learning influences. This neuromatrix model can be viewed as a *diathesis–stress model*, according to which predispositional factors interact with an acute stressor, such as pain. Once pain is established, it becomes a stressor in its own right.

The neuromatrix model of pain integrates a great deal of physiological and psychological evidence. Although the various components of the theory, as well as the theory itself, still require a considerable amount of systematic investigation, it offers another promising way of conceptualizing pain. It should stimulate a great deal of clinical research in the future.

Turk and Monarch (2002) summarized some of the main elements of the neuromatrix model:

- Pain is a multidimensional experience that is initially produced by a characteristic pattern of nerve impulses generated by a widespread neural network, or *neuromatrix*.
- Although this neuromatrix may be genetically determined to some extent, it can also be modified by sensory experiences and learning.
- When an organism is injured, there is an alteration and disruption of homeostatic regulation. Such a disruption is stressful, and it initiates a complex response of the hypothalamic–pituitary–adrenal axis, which is the body's attempt to restore homeostasis.
- Any prolonged stress, and the ongoing efforts to restore homeostasis, can subsequently suppress the immune system as well as activate the limbic system. The limbic system has an important role in emotion, motivation, and cognitive processes.

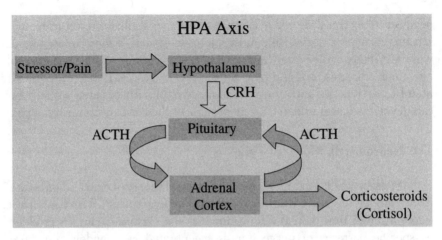

Figure 1.2. The hypothalamic–pituitary–adrenal (HPA) axis and stress. CRH = corticotrophin-releasing hormone; ACTH = adrenocorticotropic hormone.

- Once pain is established, it becomes a stressor in its own right as the body continues in its attempt to return to homeostasis; the presence of pain is a continual threat that further creates demands on the body. Fear, anxiety about the future, and the meaning of the pain contribute to the ongoing stress, thereby producing additional deviation from homeostasis. In this way, a vicious cycle develops that continues to contribute to and maintain the pain–stress process.
- According to Melzack (1999), an individual's unique neuromatrix (based on genetics as well as on interpretive sensory experiences and past learning) is the primary determinant of whether the organism experiences pain. It is also the basis for any individual differences in the pain experience.

In terms of the pain–stress cycle, Melzack (1999) pointed out that the hypothalamus stimulates corticotrophin-releasing hormone, which in turn causes the pituitary gland to release adrenocorticotropic hormone and other substances (Figure 1.2). Adrenocorticotropic hormone then stimulates the adrenal cortex to release cortisol (one of the so-called "stress hormones"). Prolonged stress means a prolonged release of cortisol. To ensure enough glucose to fuel the demand for cortisol during stress, there is a breakdown of protein in new muscle and an inhibition of the ongoing replacement of calcium in bones. This is one of the reasons why many chronic-pain conditions are characterized by muscle and joint pain.

Again, it is quite useful to educate patients about basic mechanisms of pain. To help them develop a better understanding of the relationship

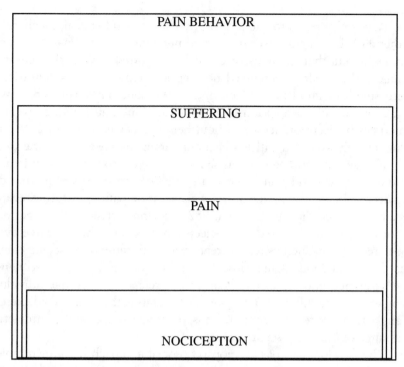

Figure 1.3. A biopsychosocial conceptual model of pain.

between stress and pain, health care professionals should provide them with a brief review of it (see Appendix 1.3).

The Biopsychosocial Perspective of Pain

Both the gate-control theory and the neuromatrix model have attempted to integrate a great deal of psychological and physiological scientific data. Although both require investigation, they highlight the most promising approach to understanding pain: the biopsychosocial approach. Indeed, the biopsychosocial model of pain, which I discuss in greater detail in chapter 2, is now accepted as the most heuristic approach to the understanding and treatment of pain disorders. It views physical disorders such as pain as a result of a complex and dynamic interaction among physiologic, psychologic, and social factors that perpetuate and may worsen the clinical presentation. Each individual experiences pain uniquely. The range of psychological, social, and economic factors can interact with physical pathology to modulate a patient's report of symptoms and subsequent disability. In fact, Loeser (1982) originally formulated a model outlining four dimensions associated with the concept of pain (see Figure 1.3): (a) nociception, (b) pain, (c) suffering, and (d) pain behavior.

Nociception refers to the actual physical units (chemical, mechanical, or thermal) that might affect specialized nerve fibers and signal the central nervous system that an aversive event has occurred. *Pain* is the sensation arising as the result of perceived nociception. However, this definition is overly simplistic and less than certain, because sometimes pain is perceived in the absence of nociception (e.g., phantom limb pain) and, conversely, sometimes nociception occurs without being perceived (e.g., an individual being severely wounded without becoming immediately aware of the pain).

Nociception and pain act as signals to the central nervous system. In contrast, *suffering* and *pain behavior* are reactions to these signals that can be affected by past experiences as well as anticipation of future events. Specifically, according to Loeser (1982), *suffering* refers to the emotional responses that are triggered by nociception or some other aversive event associated with it, such as fear, threat, or loss. Because of a specific painful episode, the individual may lose his or her job and, as a consequence, develop anxiety and depression. *Pain behavior* refers to things that individuals do when they are suffering or in pain. For example, they may avoid exercise or any activity for fear of reinjury. Thus, there may be a complex interaction of a range of biopsychosocial factors.

The development of this biopsychosocial approach has grown rapidly during the last 10 years, and in this short time a great deal of scientific knowledge has been produced concerning the best care of individuals with complex pain problems as well as pain prevention and coping techniques. As Turk and Monarch (2002) discussed in their comprehensive review of the biopsychosocial perspective on chronic pain, individuals differ significantly in how frequently they report physical symptoms, their tendency to visit physicians when experiencing identical symptoms, and their responses to the same treatments. Quite frequently, the nature of a patient's response to treatment has little to do with his or her objective physical condition. For example, White, Williams, and Greenberg (1961) earlier noted that less than one third of all individuals with clinically significant symptoms consult a physician. On the other hand, 30% to 50% of patients who seek treatment in primary care do not have specific diagnosable disorders (Dworkin & Massoth, 1994).

DISEASE VERSUS ILLNESS

Turk and Monarch (2002) went on to make the distinction between *disease* and *illness* in better understanding chronic pain. The term *disease* is generally used to define "an objective biological event" that involves the disruption of specific body structures or organ systems caused by either anatomical, pathological, or physiological changes. *Illness,* in contrast, is generally defined as a "subjective experience or self-attribution" that a disease is present. An illness will yield physical discomfort, behavioral limitations, and psychosocial distress. Thus, illness references how a sick individual and members of his or her family live with, and respond to, symptoms and disability. This distinction between disease and illness is analogous to the distinction made between pain and nociception. As noted earlier, nociception involves the stimulation of nerves that convey information about tissue damage to the brain. Pain, on the other hand, is a more subjective perception that is the result of the transduction, transmission, and modulation of sensory input. This input may be filtered through an individual's genetic composition, prior learning history, current physiological status, and sociocultural influences. Pain, therefore, cannot be comprehensively assessed without a full understanding of the person who is exposed to the nociception. The biopsychosocial model focuses on illness, which is the result of the complex interaction of biological, psychological, and social factors. With this perspective, a diversity in pain or illness expression (including its severity, duration, and psychosocial consequences) can be expected. The interrelationships among biological changes, psychological status, and the social and cultural context all need to be taken into account in fully understanding the pain patient's perception of and response to illness. A model or treatment approach that focuses on only one of these core sets of factors will be incomplete—indeed, the treatment effectiveness of a biopsychosocial approach to pain has consistently demonstrated the heuristic value of this model (Turk & Monarch, 2002).

One important postulate of the above disease-versus-illness distinction is that pain, as an illness, cannot usually be cured but only *managed*. This is also true for other chronic medical conditions, such as hypertension, diabetes, asthma, and so on. Moreover, a major current trend in the pain management literature is a movement away from the "homogeneity of pain patients myth" and toward attempts to match treatment to specific assessment outcomes of patients (e.g., Turk & Gatchel, 1999; Turk & Monarch, 2002; Turk & Okifuji, 2001). Because groups of patients may differ in psychosocial and behavioral characteristics, even when the medical diagnosis is identical, patient differences and treatment matching are important considerations. Patients with the same medical diagnosis or set of symptoms (e.g., chronic back pain, fibromyalgia, neuropathic pain) have traditionally been lumped together and then treated in the same way, as though "one size fits all." However, it has been shown that pain patients with the same diagnosis have differential responses to the same treatment. Thus, it is important that treatment be individually tailored for each patient on the basis of a careful biopsychosocial assessment of that particular patient. It is often the case that two patients experiencing chronic lower back pain, for example, will require slightly different treatment programs because of differences in their physical, psychosocial, or socioeconomic presentations. Turk and Okifuji (2001) provided a comprehensive review of the importance of this treatment-matching process and the literature that supports the greater clinical efficacy of such a strategy. Indeed, taking the approach of delineating homogeneous subgroups among patients with pain will provide an extremely important basis for the development of more specific, optimal treatment regimens for these different subgroups of patients. I discuss this approach in greater detail later in this book.

SUMMARY

In this chapter, I have provided a broad historical overview of the evolution of pain management. Today, pain is still a pervasive and costly medical problem. There is now a mandate from the Joint Commission on the Accreditation of Healthcare Organizations requiring that physicians consider pain a fifth vital sign (added to pulse, blood pressure, core body temperature, and respiration). With the Pain Care Bill of Rights of the nonprofit American Pain Foundation, there is a new zeitgeist calling for appropriate management of all types of pain, malignant and nonmalignant. There has also been a major paradigm shift in the assessment and management of pain, moving away from a traditional biomedical reductionist approach to a more comprehensive biopsychosocial approach that views physical disorders, such as pain, as a result of complex and dynamic interaction among physiologic, psychologic, and social factors that perpetuates and may even worsen the clinical presentation. An important distinction between disease and illness in better understanding pain is an integral part of the biopsychosocial perspective (Turk & Monarch, 2002). *Disease* is generally used to define an objective biological event that involves the disruption of specific body structures or organ systems caused by either anatomical, pathological, or physical changes. *Illness*, in contrast, is generally defined as a subjective experience or self-attribution that a disease is present. An illness yields physical discomfort, behavioral limitations, and psychosocial distress. The biopsychosocial model focuses on illness, which is the result of the complex interaction of biological, psychological, and social factors. In the next chapter, I discuss this biopsychosocial model of pain in greater detail.

REFERENCES

Bonica, J. J. (1953). *The management of pain.* Philadelphia: Lea & Febiger.

Dworkin, S. F., & Massoth, D. L. (1994). Temporomandibular disorders and chronic pain: Disease or illness? *Journal of Prosthetic Dentistry, 72,* 29–38.

Gatchel, R. J. (1999). Perspectives on pain: A historical overview. In R. J. Gatchel & D. C. Turk (Eds.), *Psychosocial factors in pain: Critical perspectives* (pp. 3–17). New York: Guilford Press.

Gatchel, R. J., & Turk, D. C. (1996). *Psychological approaches to pain management: A practitioner's handbook.* New York: Guilford Press.

Gatchel, R. J., & Weisberg, J. N. (2000). *Personality characteristics of patients with pain.* Washington, DC: American Psychological Association.

Joint Commission on Accreditation of Healthcare Organizations. (2000). *Pain assessment and management: An organizational approach.* Oakbrook, IL: Author.

Joranson, D. E., & Lietman, R. (1994). *The McNeil National Pain Survey.* New York: Louis Harris.

Loeser, J. D. (1982). Concepts of pain. In J. Stanton-Hicks & R. Boaz (Eds.), *Chronic low back pain* (pp. 109–142). New York: Raven Press.

Loeser, J. D. (2003). The decade of pain control and research. *APS Bulletin, 13,* 5.

Marketdata Enterprises. (2001). *Chronic pain management clinics: A market analysis.* Tampa, FL: Author.

Melzack, R. (1993). Pain: Past, present and future. *Canadian Journal of Experimental Psychology, 47,* 615–629.

Melzack, R. (1999). Pain and stress: A new perspective. In R. J. Gatchel & D. C. Turk (Eds.), *Psychosocial factors in pain: Critical perspectives* (pp. 89–106). New York: Guilford Press.

Melzack, R., & Wall, P. D. (1965). Pain mechanisms: A new theory. *Science, 50,* 971–979.

Nathan, P. W. (1976). The gate control theory of pain: A critical review. *Brain, 99,* 123–158.

National Research Council. (2001). *Musculoskeletal disorders and the workplace: Low back and upper extremities.* Washington, DC: National Academy Press.

Pleis, J. R., & Coles, R. (1998). Summary health statistics for U.S. adults: National Health Interview Survey, 1998. *National Center for Health Statistics, Vital Health Statistics, 202*(10), 209.

Schweitzer, A. (1922). *On the edge of the primeval forest.* Baltimore: Johns Hopkins University Press.

Selye, H. (1950). *Stress.* Montreal, Quebec, Canada: Acta Medical Publishers.

Turk, D. C., & Gatchel, R. J. (1999). Psychosocial factors and pain: Revolution and evolution. In R. J. Gatchel & D. C. Turk (Eds.), *Psychosocial factors in pain: Critical perspectives.* New York: Guilford Press.

Turk, D. C., & Monarch, E. S. (2002). Biopsychosocial perspective on chronic pain. In D. C. Turk & R. J. Gatchel (Eds.), *Psychological approaches to pain management: A practitioner's handbook* (2nd ed., pp. 3–29). New York: Guilford Press.

Turk, D. C., & Okifuji, A. (2001). Matching treatment to assessment of patients with chronic pain. In D. C. Turk & R. Melzack (Eds.), *Handbook of pain assessment* (2nd ed., pp. 400–414). New York: Guilford Press.

U.S. Bureau of the Census. (1996). *Statistical abstract of the United States: 1996* (116th ed.). Washington, DC: Author.

Wall, P. D. (1989). The dorsal horn. In P. D. Wall & R. Melzack (Eds.), *Textbook of pain* (2nd ed., pp. 102–111). New York: Churchill Livingstone.

White, K. L., Williams, F., & Greenberg, B. G. (1961). The etiology of medical care. *New England Journal of Medicine, 265,* 885–886.

APPENDIX 1.1

Recommended Readings

Gatchel, R. J. (1999). Perspectives on pain: A historical overview. In R. J. Gatchel & D. C. Turk (Eds.), *Psychosocial factors in pain: Critical perspectives* (pp. 3–17). New York: Guilford Press.

Lechnyr, R., & Lechnyr, T. (2003). The psychological dimension of pain management. *Practical Pain Management, 3,* 10–18.

Turk, D. C., & Monarch, E. S. (2002). Biopsychosocial perspective on chronic pain. In D. C. Turk & R. J. Gatchel (Eds.), *Psychological approaches to pain management: A practitioner's handbook* (2nd ed., pp. 3–29). New York: Guilford Press.

APPENDIX 1.2

The American Pain Foundation's Pain Care Bill of Rights

As a Person with Pain, You Have:

- The right to have your report of pain taken seriously and to be treated with dignity and respect by doctors, nurses, pharmacists, and other healthcare professionals.
- The right to have your pain thoroughly assessed and promptly treated.
- The right to be informed by your doctor about what may be causing your pain, possible treatments, and the benefits, risks and costs of each.
- The right to participate actively in decisions about how to manage your pain.
- The right to have your pain reassessed regularly and your treatment adjusted if your pain has not been eased.
- The right to be referred to a pain specialist if your pain persists.
- The right to get clear and prompt answers to your questions, take time to make decisions, and refuse a particular type of treatment if you choose.

Although not always required by law, these are the rights you should expect, and if necessary demand, for your pain care.

For more information, contact the American Pain Foundation, 201 North Charles Street, Suite 710, Baltimore, MD 21201-4111, or visit http://www.painfoundation.org. To review current legislation related to pain issues, visit the "Thomas" government Web site (in the spirit of Thomas Jefferson): http://thomas.loc.gov/.

APPENDIX 1.3

What Is Stress?

Stress may represent the single most significant threat to physical and emotional health we face today. Medical statistics suggest that as much as 80% of present-day diseases may have their origin in stress. Stress is an everyday fact of life; you cannot avoid it. You experience stress from three sources: (a) your environment, (b) your body, and (c) your thoughts. Your environment bombards you with demands to adjust. You must learn to endure and adapt to noise, traffic, crowding, time deadlines, financial pressure, and interpersonal demands. Your body is affected by illness, injury, diet, and drugs, as well as by environmental events (e.g., the death of a family member, job change). Your reaction to stress is very much influenced by an innate fight-or-flight response that all people have. The fight-or-flight response is activated when your environment is perceived as threatening or dangerous. It prepares you to flee from danger or fight if necessary. Unfortunately, most of the stress we face today cannot be overcome by fleeing or fighting. Instead, we must learn to control this fight-or-flight response in different ways. This is what this treatment program is all about.

A person experiencing stress will notice changes in one or more of three different systems: (a) physical responses, (b) thoughts, and (c) behaviors. Physical responses of stress may include increased breathing rate, muscular tension in your face and jaw, increased heart rate, nausea or diarrhea, sweating, and so on. Thoughts associated with stress include a sense of impending catastrophe, worrying, a sense of helplessness, and so on. The resulting behaviors include diminished performance and restlessness and fidgeting and may even lead to avoidance of certain situations associated with the stress. Stress will also affect your pain. The more stress you experience, the more likely that your pain will become worse.

Think about your body as being like a car and your nervous system as like a car engine. When you drive your car, you have to speed up and slow down with the flow of traffic. Your car engine rests on idle when you come up to a stoplight, but it revs up high when you get onto the highway. Just like a car engine, your nervous system speeds up and slows down during the day, depending on what you are doing, thinking, and feeling and what is going on around you. Most of the time you don't even notice increases and decreases in the stress level in your body. Fluctuations in the stress level in your body are normal and healthy.

When you have a lot of stressful things going on in your life, then the stress level in your body can remain too high. Emotions such as anxiety, worry, anger, and depression can produce stress chemicals in your body and keep your internal engine revved up. When the stress in your body remains too high for too long, then things inside your body can start to wear out.

This can cause physical symptoms (e.g., muscle tension, headaches, acid stomach, fatigue, and high blood pressure). When stress remains too high for long enough, heart attacks and strokes may result.

Again, think about the car engine. The more stress you put on a car engine, the more quickly the engine parts will wear out. Probably the weaker parts will wear out first. Just like the car engine, the weakest systems in your body will tend to be affected first by stress and may wear out. Different people's bodies react to stress in different ways. Some people get headaches, some get stomachaches, some get high blood pressure. Probably your injured body area is one of your weaker parts now. Your pain level is probably one of the first things that can be affected when your stress level is too high for too long.

You can have a high level of stress in your body without even knowing it. In fact, most people have some stress and tension in their bodies of which they are not aware. You can become more aware of the stress level in your body, and you can learn how to reduce your stress by practicing relaxation exercises and participating in biofeedback training.

The Pain–Stress Cycle

The pain–stress cycle plays a key role in understanding how your feelings and behaviors affect pain. Interventions at any point in the cycle affect other parts of the cycle. If pain is lowered, then stress and worry decrease. If stress and worry are lowered, then pain is decreased. Pain, stress, and worry are related, and a change in one affects the others. Stress, tension, or worry can increase pain intensity and decrease a person's pain threshold. Many people who have persistent pain find themselves stuck in a cycle of feeling stress, increasing tension, and pain. In understanding how your behaviors are contributing to your pain–stress–tension cycle, you can gain more control over your pain.

Treatment for Stress

A number of research studies have shown that individuals can control their stress by learning to relax their bodies and thinking in a more rational manner. People learn to be tense, and they can learn to relax. Learning to relax is like learning any new skill; it takes place gradually and only after regular practice. A treatment program can teach you a number of skills to help you control your stress and tension.

2

THE BIOPSYCHOSOCIAL
APPROACH TO PAIN
ASSESSMENT AND MANAGEMENT

To heal does not necessarily imply to cure. It can simply mean helping to achieve a way of life compatible with their individual aspirations— to restore their freedom to make choices—even in the presence of continuing disease.

—Rene Dubos (1978)

In this chapter, I review the biopsychosocial approach to pain assessment and management. Indeed, as I discussed in chapter 1, the biopsychosocial model is now viewed as the most heuristic approach; it appropriately conceptualizes pain as a complex and dynamic interaction among physiologic, psychologic, and social factors that often results in, or at least maintains, pain. It cannot be broken down into distinct, independent psychosocial or physical components. Each individual also experiences pain uniquely. The complexity of pain is especially evident when it persists over time, as a range of psychological, social, and economic factors can interact with physical pathology to modulate a patient's report of pain and subsequent disability. The model uses physiologic, biologic, cognitive, emotional, behavioral, and social factors, as well as their interplay, when explaining a patient's report of pain.

There is currently a revolution in developing a more comprehensive, biopsychosocial understanding of pain. Besides the greater appreciation of psychosocial factors that contribute to the pain process, there is a growing understanding of how endocrine modulation of pain mechanisms occurs. Also, research on pain mechanisms and pathways has greatly expanded in scope during the past few years, including the use of a wide array of techniques, such as anatomical, electrophysiological, genetic, molecular biological, and pharmacological approaches. Technical advances have also improved methods for identifying brain regions involved in various neurological and psychiatric conditions. This synergy across disciplines will, it is hoped, lead to the most effective methods to manage pain, because it will help researchers understand how the nervous system senses, interprets, and responds to pain (Gatchel, 1999).

Turk and Monarch (2002) provided a comprehensive review of the biopsychosocial perspective on chronic pain. Earlier, Turk (1999) also indicated that, within a biopsychosocial context, pain problems need to be "viewed longitudinally as ongoing, multifactorial processes in which there is a dynamic and reciprocal interplay among biological, psychological, and social cultural factors that shapes the experience in responses of patients" (p. 20). Thus, to comprehensively assess pain, one must be sure to account for such potential interactions before prescribing the best treatment regimen, individualized for a particular patient with pain. For example, a patient may present with chronic pain resulting from an earlier accident, which produced severe musculoskeletal injuries, such as bone fractures and ligament tears that have not completely healed. Besides these physical injuries and resultant pain, the accident may have led to the inability to work again. The patient might also have self-esteem problems because he or she is viewed as being disabled and is stigmatized by it. This may have also resulted in economic problems and stressors because of the sudden decrease in income. There are debts to be paid, causing family stress, turmoil, and guilt. If this patient comes from a "macho" culture in which work and activity are highly valued, there may be even more psychosocial distress. Thus, as one can see, there are potentially multiple levels of psychosocial issues that all need to be assessed before one can develop a comprehensive pain management program for a patient such as this (see Figure 2.1). One may need to assess the patient individually, as well as in the context of the family, workplace, and other social situations. This is not an example of an atypical chronic-pain patient; it is more the norm than the exception.

PAIN, DISABILITY, AND IMPAIRMENT

Before I review the methods to assess and manage pain, it is very important to become aware of the vagaries and difficulties inherent in differentiating among the constructs of *pain*, *disability*, and *impairment*. This is because there is frequently a discordance among the levels of pain, disability, and impairment displayed by a patient. Such discordance often creates major problems for assessment and treatment personnel when selecting the best goal for developing a therapeutic plan and indexing therapeutic progress.

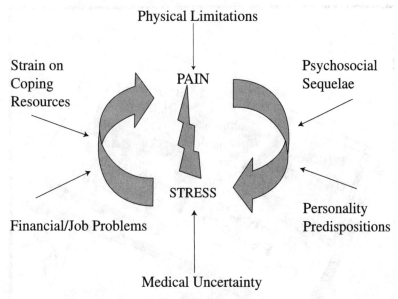

Physical Limitations

Strain on
Coping
Resources

PAIN

Psychosocial
Sequelae

STRESS

Financial/Job Problems

Personality
Predispositions

Medical Uncertainty

Figure 2.1. The pain–stress cycle, emphasizing the interaction of stress-related issues and the actual pain. It is helpful to draw patients' attention to this cycle. From "How Practitioners Should Evaluate Personality to Help Manage Patients With Chronic Pain," by R. J. Gatchel, in *Personality Characteristics of Patients With Pain*, edited by R. J. Gatchel and J. N. Weisberg, 2000, Washington, DC: American Psychological Association. Copyright 2000 by the American Psychological Association. Reprinted with permission.

Indeed, Waddell (1987) originally indicated that, although correlations are found among these phenomena (usually in the range of .6), overlap among these categories is not perfect. As can be seen in Figure 2.2, although these factors are all logically and clinically overlapping, there is usually not a 1:1:1 relationship among them. What makes this imperfect correlation even more complex is the wide range of individual differences in such discordance

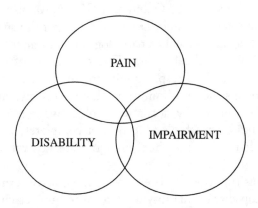

PAIN

DISABILITY

IMPAIRMENT

Figure 2.2. Discordance among levels of pain, impairment, and disability.

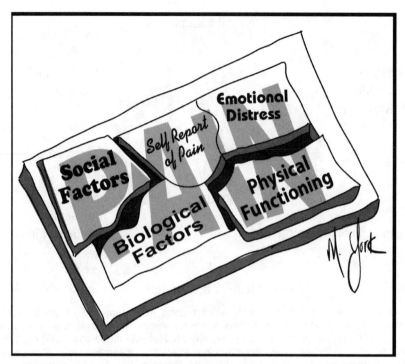

The biopsychosocial perspective of pain emphasizing the interaction of biological and psychosocial factors in understanding pain.

from one patient to the next. Therefore, health care professionals need to be aware of the varying relationships among these constructs. Turk and Melzack (2001) also noted this potential complexity.

Clinicians should also be aware of the definitions of these three constructs or concepts, because they are fundamentally different. These terms have been discussed in the medical impairment and disability evaluation literature (e.g., Dembe, 2000; Gatchel, 1996). *Impairment* is a physical/ medical term that refers to an alteration of the patient's usual health status (i.e., some objective anatomical or pathological abnormality) that is evaluated by physical and medical means. The evaluation of impairment has traditionally been a medical responsibility in which there is an attempt to objectively evaluate structural limitations. Unfortunately, current technology does not allow a totally accurate or objective physical impairment evaluation; it relies on methods that are not completely reliable, that are sometimes subject to examiner bias, and that are not yet associated with good diagnostic validity.

Disability has traditionally been an administrative term that refers to the diminished capacity or inability to perform certain activities of everyday living; it is the resulting loss of function due to impairment. Disability evaluations, too, are often not totally reliable and are subject to various examiner and patient response biases. The assessment of disability is usually based on subjective self-report measures of restrictions of activities of daily living, such as walking, sleep, work and recreational activities, sex, and so on. Finally, *pain* is a psychophysiologic concept based primarily on an experiential or subjective evaluation. It is also quite often difficult to quantify objectively in a reliable manner.

Although physical impairment, disability, and pain can be separately assessed, they are not highly correlated. One patient may verbally report a significant amount of pain but show little impairment that can be objectively evaluated, with disability perhaps lying somewhere between the two in severity. Another patient may report little pain but display great disability and some impairment. Consequently, it is extremely important to assess all three constructs in specific situations whenever possible, with the expectation that there may be complex interactions among them that may differ from one patient to the next, as well as from one time to the next.

What complicates the above issue even more is the fact that there are three broad categories of measures—physical, psychological, and overt behavior/function (i.e., observable behaviors such as walking, lifting, bending, etc.)—that have all been used to assess patients. However, again, these three major measurement categories (or biopsychosocial referents) may not always display high concordance with one another when measuring a construct such as pain or disability. It has long been noted in the psychology literature, for example, that self-report, overt behavior, and physiological indexes of a construct such as pain or stress sometime show low correlations among one another (e.g., Gatchel, 2000). Therefore, if one uses a self-report measure as a primary index of a construct such as pain, and compares it to the overt behavioral or physiologic index of the same construct, direct overlap cannot automatically be expected. Moreover, two different self-report indexes or physiological indexes of the same construct may not be as highly correlated as one would desire (see Figure 2.3). What has plagued the evaluation arena in general has been the lack of agreement in the wide variation of measures used to document constructs such as pain, disability, and impairment, as well as changes in these constructs. Therefore, the literature is replete with many different measurement techniques and tests of a construct such as pain. However, the literature is beginning to demonstrate which measures appear to be the most reliable and valid (Gatchel, 2001). Indeed, as Tukey (1979) noted:

> When the right thing can only be measured poorly, it tends to cause the wrong thing to be measured well. And it is often much worse to have a good measurement of the wrong thing—especially when, as is so often the case, the wrong thing will IN FACT be used as an indicator

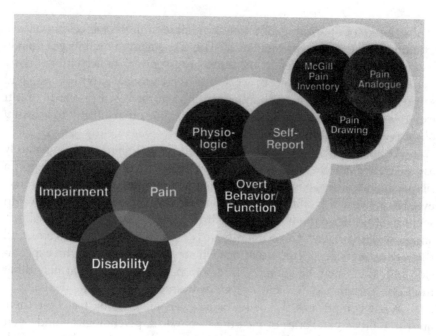

Figure 2.3. The often-low concordance among and within physical, psychosocial, and overt behavior/function measures. From "Research Alert," by R. J. Gatchel, *APS Bulletin, 8*(4), p. 26. Copyright 1998 by R. J. Gatchel. Reprinted with permission.

of the right thing—than to have a poor measurement of the right thing. (p. 788)

With the above quotation in mind, it is very important to avoid many pitfalls often encountered when attempting to measure the *right thing* with *good measurements*. A number of recent works provide comprehensive reviews of "good measurements" of pain, for example, Gatchel (2001), Gatchel and Weisberg (2000), and Turk and Melzack (2001). Of course, when using a particular test or measurement approach, one must be aware of the instrument's psychometric properties. Jensen (2003) provided an excellent review of such properties. This is important, because if a health care professional uses a particular test or measurement, he or she will have to defend its use. The basic way of defending it is to cite literature that has demonstrated that the instrument has good psychometric properties. Two core psychometric properties are reliability and validity. *Reliability* refers to the reproducibility of a test from one administration to the next. One would expect that if a test is administered at two points in time, with no major intervening circumstances possibly affecting the construct or dimension one is measuring (e.g., intelligence level or personality), then the test–retest reliability should be high. If not, there may be flaws in the test that make it less than acceptable for use.

Validity refers to the appropriateness and usefulness of a particular test or measurement in making an inference about an individual's behavior (e.g., the level of pain being experienced). If a test was designed to measure pain, then it should tap that quality. There are, in turn, different types of validity:

- *Predictive validity* refers to whether test scores can predict subsequent measures or behaviors. For example, will a high score on Pain Test A predict whether a patient will require a greater amount of pain management?
- *Concurrent validity* refers to whether test scores are correlated with other current measures or behaviors. For example, is a high score on Pain Test A correlated with the amount of pain medication a patient is now taking, or to his or her level of activities of daily living, and so on?
- *Content validity* refers to whether test scores are representative of the quality being measured. This is usually evaluated by having, say, experts in the field of pain agree that a measure or test of pain is actually evaluating that quality.
- *Construct validity* is somewhat abstract and difficult to define. A *construct* is a theoretical phenomenon, such as anxiety, pain, intelligence, temperament, and so on. Construct validity is concerned with the extent to which a test relates to some objective behavior, as well as to the particular theoretical model at hand. Because of this two-way relationship between theory and practice, construct validity is actually a process. It serves both as a check on theory and as a spur to the same theory. For example, for the construct of pain, the theorist seeks to develop a measure of pain. Lacking a specific criterion, however, the theorist may have to use certain behaviors as indicators of pain (e.g., self-report, grimacing, inability to work, pain medication use, etc.). It may then be possible to formulate and test hypotheses about how pain, as it is measured on a test, does or does not relate to other behaviors in particular situations. On the basis of the findings, the theorist then progressively revises and refines the construct. Construct validation, therefore, involves systematically testing and revising hypotheses about a construct by examining the empirically found relationships among responses in different situations. It is a form of hypothesis testing and theory building.

Health care professionals need to constantly remain up to date in terms of what assessment measures and tests have the best psychometric properties. A regular review of the clinical research literature will help in this process. Again, if tests are used, then the clinician will be called on to defend them by insurance companies, the judicial system, and so on. If the health care professional cannot stay up to date in regard to assessment measures, they can be brought up to the state's ethics board for providing a poor assessment and inappropriately billing for it.

It should also be pointed out that there are two important "assumption traps" that pain management professionals need to avoid when considering the best assessment measure to use. First, one cannot automatically assume, on an a priori basis, that one assessment measure will necessarily be more valid or reliable than another. In general, the more objectively quantified the measure is, the more likely it can be empirically established as a valid and reliable referent or marker. The second assumption trap is that a physical measure will always be more objective than self-report psychosocial measures. However, regardless of the level of accuracy or sophistication of a mechanical device used in collecting physiologic measures, it is always the case that human interpretation must be used in the understanding of the resulting findings. In addition, it must be remembered that a patient's performance during a physical assessment protocol can be greatly influenced by fear of pain or injury, motivation, instructional set, and so on (Gatchel, 2001).

Finally, the new International Association for the Study of Pain Core Curriculum, 3rd revision, now delineates a number of important concepts that should be taught to pain assessment and management specialists concerning disability and functional and psychiatric assessment (see Exhibit 2.1).

PAIN ASSESSMENT TECHNIQUES

At the outset, as noted earlier, the common denominator of all assessment methods is the qualities of validity, reliability (reproducibility), and predictive value (e.g., Anderrson, Pope, Frymoyer, & Snook, 1991). However, there often remain frequent misunderstandings over the appropriate use of assessments based on the generalizability of the scientific reports or validity to the circumstances in which the health care professional is using the assessment method. Such ambiguities can be minimized by examining the match between the clinical context in which a test is evaluated and the patient to whom it is applied in the clinical setting. Basically, one must answer the question of a test's validity by addressing "valid for what?" Assessment methods may be valid for measuring specific biologic/physiologic states but have no validity in predicting, for example, impairment, disability, or activities of daily living. Moreover, the results of the test may or may not be valid for informing or clarifying treatment planning. With this caveat in mind, I discuss next the various potential assessment approaches that can be used with patients experiencing pain. Of course, readers must keep in mind that, when embracing a comprehensive biopsychosocial assessment model, it

EXHIBIT 2.1
Important Concepts That Should Be Taught to
Pain Assessment and Management Specialists

- Understand the distinction and interrelationship among chronic pain, impairment, disability, and incapacity for work.
- Understand the different epidemiology of chronic pain, health care usage, and associated disability and incapacity for work.
- Understand the musculoskeletal, soft tissue, and neurophysiologic bases of chronic pain and the methods and limitations of assessing them clinically in the individual patient.
- Understand the role of psychologic, behavioral, and social factors in chronic pain, disability, and (in)capacity for work and the methods and limitations of assessing them clinically in the individual patient.
- Understand the possible influence of workers' compensation and litigation on the clinical presentation, evaluation, and management outcomes of chronic pain.
- Understand occupational health issues in chronic pain, disability, and (in)capacity for work. Understand the concepts, methods, and limitations of yellow flags, barriers to recovery, rehabilitation and return-to-work interventions.
- Understand the different disability systems and the different approaches to disability evaluation. Understand the need for a systematic approach to the assessment of disability and (in)capacity, the application of test results, and the preparation of a report directed to the particular referral question.
- Understand the role and limitations of medical and psychological/psychiatric evidence in the workers' compensation, Social Security, and litigation systems.
- Understand the concepts, methods, and limitations of assessing chronic pain clinically in the individual patient, including the American Medical Association Guides, 5th edition.
- Understand the concepts, methods, and limitations of independent medical examinations.
- Understand the concepts, methods, and limitations of functional capacity evaluations.
- Understand the concepts, methods, and limitations of assessment of malingering, exaggeration, and credibility (including related *Diagnostic and Statistical Manual of Mental Disorders* [American Psychiatric Association, 1994] and World Health Organization definitions [1989]).

Note. From *Core Curriculum for Professional Education in Pain,* edited by J. E. Charlton, G. Gourlay, and S. H. Butler, 2005, Seattle, WA: International Association for the Study of Pain Press. Copyright 2005 by International Association of Pain. Reprinted with permission.

is important to consider each successive measure in context with the other measures to be integrated. This will lead to the most comprehensive assessment of a patient, which will then significantly contribute to the development of the best treatment regimen for dealing with the pain problem. In chapter 4 of this book, I discuss more information about this in the context of a *stepwise approach* to pain assessment. This stepwise approach to assessment proceeds from global indexes of biopsychosocial concomitants of pain to more detailed evaluations of specific diagnoses. Likewise, the *stepped-care*

EXHIBIT 2.2
Commonly Used Psychosocial Instruments for the Assessment of Patients Experiencing Pain

Beck Anxiety Inventory
Beck Depression Inventory—II
Chronic Pain Coping Inventory
Clinical Observational Technique of Pain Behavior
Coping Strategies Questionnaire
Fear Avoidance Beliefs Questionnaire
McGill Pain Questionnaire
Million Visual Analogue Scale
Millon Behavioral Health Inventory
Millon Behavioral Medicine Diagnostic
Minnesota Multiphasic Personality Inventory—2
Multidimensional Pain Inventory
Oswestry Pain Disability Questionnaire
Pain Disability Questionnaire
Quantify Pain Drawing
Roland and Morris Disability Questionnaire
SF-36 Health Survey
Sickness Impact Profile
Symptom Checklist–90, Revised
Ways of Coping Questionnaire—Revised

framework for managing pain in a primary-care setting is presented in chapter 5 as well as extended for use in secondary- and tertiary-care settings.

A Review of Commonly Used Instruments for Pain Assessment

Some of the commonly used psychosocial instruments for the assessment of patients experiencing pain are presented in Exhibit 2.2. Keep in mind that no one type of assessment measure can usually capture all the important characteristics when considering a patient's report of pain; rather, the integration of a number of assessment tools is needed. A more thorough description of these instruments can be found in Gatchel (2001) and Turk and Melzack (2001).

Medical/Biopsychosocial Evaluation

Pain is a cardinal symptom of disease; however, pain sometimes does not fit neatly into an evaluative–curative model of medical care. From a biopsychosocial perspective, evaluation of pain should include a medical history, physical examination, and appropriate medical tests, as well as psychosocial assessment. Indeed, several important organizations in the

United States have recently developed new standards for the evaluation of pain. As noted in chapter 1, pain is now considered the fifth vital sign. The Joint Commission on Accreditation of Healthcare Organizations therefore requires that pain severity be documented using a pain scale. In addition, patients' own words to describe their pain, pain location, duration, aggravating and alleviating factors, present pain management regimen and effectiveness, the effects of pain, the patient's pain goal, and a physical examination, are all to be documented during the initial assessment (Joint Commission on Accreditation of Healthcare Organizations, 2000). In chapter 1, Exhibit 1.1 presented an example of how to accomplish these requirements.

The Health Care Financing Administration also has standards for medical evaluations that have relevance for pain evaluations of patients whose care is governed within Medicare standards. A review of the documentation's standards is highly recommended for providers using evaluation and management codes for patients in the Medicare system. The patient's chief complaint must be documented and, depending on the level of service for the evaluation, one to four additional historical items must be documented. These may include pain location, severity, quality, duration, timing, context, modifying factors, and associated signs and symptoms. Documentation requirements for past medical history, family history, and social history are required when pertinent, except for the higher levels of service, which require documentation of a finding for each of the following three categories: (a) *past medical history*, (b) *family history*, and (c) *social history*. It is clear that medications, allergies, surgeries related to pain, medical (including psychiatric or psychological) diagnosis, past treatments for pain, family history of pain, history of substance abuse, disability, litigation, psychosocial stressors, and other patient-specific information of past family and social history are important. Physical examination documentation guidelines are too complicated to summarize here, but a number of physical findings that count toward satisfying documentation requirements are as follows:

- A slow respiratory rate and small pupils may indicate the presence of opioids.
- Reduced peripheral impulses may be a sign of peripheral vascular disease, especially in patients with pain in the same extremity.
- Gait and posture should be examined.
- The patient's range of motion and instability should be assessed.
- Muscle strength should be evaluated.
- As part of a neurologic examination, cranial nerve reflexes, sensation, and coordination should be assessed.
- Speech, thought processes, associations, judgment orientation, recent remote memory, attention span and concentration, language, mood, and affect should be inspected.

The Commission on Accreditation of Rehabilitation Facilities (2001) also developed new guidelines for the assessment of patients with pain who are candidates for rehabilitation programs. This requires not only a medical evaluation but also evaluation of patient functioning; physical assessment; psychosocial assessment; social and vocational assessments; and, when indicated, a spirituality referral. It requires that the participants in the assessment are the patient, the physician, and a psychologist. Additional assessments may be made by a physical therapist, an occupational therapist, a vocational specialist, a biofeedback therapist, or some combination of these. Assessment criteria for entry into a pain management rehabilitation program must be matched to predicted outcomes, frequency of service, intensity of service, and duration of service. Pediatric patients must have their family included as a part of the assessment team.

Laboratory testing for patients with diffused aches and pain include a complete blood test, including blood count; Westergreen erythrocyte sedimentation rate (a procedure for estimating the sedimentation rate of red blood cells in fluid blood); thyroid stimulating hormone, calcium; phosphorus; and, if weakness is present, creatine kinase (an enzyme-catalyzing process important in muscle contraction). As an example of such laboratory testing, a summary of rheumatological diseases is presented in Table 2.1.

When needed, radiographic evaluations should usually begin with plane film (i.e., x-rays). Flexion and extension spine plane films are frequently necessary for the evaluation of spinal instability, which is sometimes present in patients with chronic neck or back pain who have a nondiagnostic magnetic resonance imagery finding. Electrodiagnostic evaluations are also sometimes very helpful; however, caution should be exercised when multiple abnormalities exist.

Red herrings are often not uncommon in medical evaluations, especially when patients have seen multiple physicians and have had multiple tests. Indeed, several weaknesses exist regarding pain evaluations. Improvements in the ability to evaluate patients for secondary gain factors, such as patients with disability issues or pending litigation, need to be considered (I review such factors in chap. 7). Disability determinations need to be accurate and precise. This is frequently not the case and often leads to pitfalls. In addition, improvements in the ability to assess patients for substance abuse, other psychiatric disorders, or both, is needed.

Impairment Evaluation

A widely accepted definition of *impairment* is the one developed by the World Health Organization (1980): "any loss or abnormality of psychological, physiological, or anatomical structure or function" (p. 19). In the United States, the American Medical Association (Cocchiarella, 1993), in

TABLE 2.1
Summary of Testing for a Number of Rheumatological Diseases

	Autoantibody	Antigen specificity	ANA pattern	Disease associations
Nucleic acids	Anti-DNP	Deoxyribonucleoprotein	Homogeneous/peripheral	SLE, drug-induced LE
	Anti-DNA	Deoxyribonucleic acid	Homogeneous/peripheral	SLE, but also in other diseases SLE, SLE nephritis
	Double-stranded DNA			SLE, drug-induced SLE, RA, Sjögren's Syndrome
	Single-stranded DNA			SLE
	Anti-RNA	Ribonucleic acid	?	
	Anti-nucleolar	4-6s RNA, U3RNP	Nucleolar	Systemic sclerosis, SLE
Histones	Anti-histone		Homogeneous/peripheral	SLE, drug-induced LE
	Anti-histone (H3)		Large speckles	SLE
Non-histone Nuclear proteins	Anti-Sm (Anti-ENA)	Smith	Speckle	SLE
	Anti-nRNP (Anti-ENA)	Ribonucleoprotein (UIRNP)	Speckle	SLE MCTD
	Anti-SS-A/Ro		Speckle (weak)	Sjögren's syndrome SLE Subacute cutaneous LE Neonatal lupus
	Anti-SS-B/La/Ha		Fine speckle	Sjögren's syndrome SLE
	Anti-MA-1	MA-1	?	SLE
	Anti-Sc-70	Scleroderma 70	Speckle	Systemic sclerosis
	Anti-PCNA	Proliferating cell nuclear antigen	Variable speckle	SLE

(continues)

TABLE 2.1 (Continued)

	Autoantibody	Antigen specificity	ANA pattern	Disease associations
Cytoplasmic	Anti-centriole	Centriole	Large speckles	Systemic sclerosis
	Anti-Golgi	Golgi	Perinuclear strands	SLE
	Anti-mitochondria	Mitochondria	Irregular granules	SLE Primary biliary cirrhosis
	Anti-ribosomal	Ribosomes/ribonucleoprotein	Fine speckles	SLE
	Anti-vimentin	Vimentin	Large fibrils	RA, Sjögren's syndrome
	Antineutrophilic cytoplasmic antibody	Serine proteinase and myeloperoxidase		Wegener's polyarteritis nodosa, glomerulonephritis
Other	Anti-centromere	Chromosomal centromere	Discrete speckles	System sclerosis Raynaud's
	Anti-nuclear matrix	Nuclear matrix	Irregular speckles	MCTD, SLE
	Anti-Mi-1	Mi-1	?	Polymyositis (adult)
	Anti-Jo-1	Jo-1	Cytoplasm?	Polymyositis
	Anti-Ku	Ku	?	Polymyositis (adult)
	Anti-systems, A,B,C	Su (systems A, B, C)	?	Polymyositis (adult)
	Anti-Pm-1 (Pm-Scl)	PM-1 (Pm-Scl)	?	Polymyositis/systemic sclerosis overlap
	Anti-RANA	RANA	Speckles	RA

Note. DNP = deoxyribonucleoprotein; DNA = deoxyribonucleic acid; RNA = ribonucleic acid; RANA = rheumatoid arthritis associated nuclear antigen; PM-1 = polymyositis; MCTD = mixed connective tissue disease. From "Evaluation of Musculoskeletal Symptoms," by M. H. Liang and R. D. Sturrock, in *Practical Rheumatology* (p. 16), edited by J. H. Klippel and P. A. Dieppe, 1995, St. Louis, MO: Mosby. Copyright 1995 by Elsevier. Adapted with permission.

its *Guides to the Evaluation of Permanent Impairment* (4th ed.), subsequently defined *impairment* as "a decrease in, or loss or absence of, the capacity of an individual to meet personal, social, or occupational demands, or to meet statutory or regulatory requirements." The *Guides* go on to propose methods that quantify impairments associated with a wide array of medical conditions, ranging on a scale from 0% (when there is no impairment) to 100% (when an individual is completely incapacitated). It is assumed that impairment measures the medical component of disability and, furthermore, that the magnitude of a person's impairment correlates closely with the severity of his or her disadvantage in the workplace. Thus, it attempts to document not only whether a patient has an impairment but also how severe the impairment is. Dembe (2000) discussed the many complexities involved in such an impairment determination.

The *functional capacity evaluation* (FCE) is the most widely used standard method of evaluating a worker's capacity to perform vocational functions and activities. Moreover, as Matheson (1995) noted, an FCE is quite critical because it provides a standard method of translating the effect of impairment into disability (which I discuss in the next section). Indeed, FCEs can provide an objective and systematic method of estimating a person's functional capacity to perform occupational tasks. The purposes of the FCE may include the following: substantiation of impairment, determining level of disability, specifying job handicaps, establishing return-to-work limitations, establishing functional baselines at the outset of rehabilitation efforts, and providing objective monitoring or functional improvement during rehabilitation efforts. The various functions usually evaluated in an FCE include activities such as lifting, pulling, pushing, bending, sitting, climbing, and grasping. Measurements evaluated usually involve the individual's strength, lifting capacity, aerobic capacity, endurance, range of motion, manual dexterity, and other necessary indicators of work capacity for a particular individual. The reliability and validity of FCEs have been documented in a number of studies (Gatchel, 2001). Two of the most commonly used FCEs are the California Functional Capacity Protocol (Matheson, 2001) and the Employment and Rehabilitation Institute of California (ERIC) work tolerance screening battery (Matheson & Ogden, 1993).

Disability Evaluation

Robinson (2001) provided an excellent review of the complexities involved in a disability evaluation of a patient with a painful condition. Of course, the fundamental goal of the disability evaluation procedure is to ascertain whether a patient can or cannot work. However, such a determination is often quite difficult in evaluating painful conditions because of the misguided assumption that impairment (discussed in the last section of this chapter) can be precisely and objectively measured and is closely linked to "mechanical failure" of an organ or body part. However, chronic-pain patients often complain of activity restrictions that cannot be fully understood in terms of a specific mechanical failure. As I discussed earlier, there is often a low concordance between subjective reports of pain and objective data of impairment; this will thus introduce vagaries into the disability evaluation process. One disability evaluator may mostly ignore the patient's subjective reports of pain and disability and rely more heavily on any available objective evidence of mechanical dysfunction; another evaluator may rely more exclusively on the subjective appraisals and activity restrictions reported by the patient, regardless of whether they can be objectively quantified in terms of any measurable mechanical failure or dysfunction. Still another evaluator may attempt to develop a composite of both the subjective and objective measures. Unfortunately, as Robinson (2001) and Dembe (2000) have noted, there is currently no totally agreed-on disability evaluation system that can be used. Thus, disability agencies across different states will be quite different in the methods used. It should also be remembered that, across the different states, there is no one workers' compensation system; each state's workers' compensation system is specific for that state. Therefore, disability evaluations in Texas may be quite different from those in California or Connecticut. Nevertheless, in terms of a disability evaluation, physicians are usually required to address the following areas: assessment and diagnosis, impairment, ability to work, and a need for further treatment. Robinson (2001) provided examples of the questions that are usually asked by disability agencies when conducting such evaluations.

PAIN MANAGEMENT TECHNIQUES

Woessner (2003) appropriately pointed out that the treatment approaches used often depend on the broad diagnosed source(s) of pain. He delineated three major diagnostic sources that are useful to keep in mind when assessing pain and then developing a treatment plan: (a) nociceptive pain, (b) neuropathic pain, and (c) central pain. Disease or pathophysiological processes usually will cause mechanical or chemical pain, which is often nociceptive in nature. Often, such pain is acute in nature and acts as a signal demanding attention (e.g., sprains and strains, contusions, a benign cyst, etc.). As long as central or neuropathic pain problems do not develop (because of physiological alterations of central pathways or nerve damage), then there are a number of effective acute-care treatment options available (e.g., medication, rest followed by therapeutic exercise and manual therapies).

Neuropathic pain, often the result of nerve damage, can occur via many mechanisms because pain fibers can transmit, and can also be perceived as transmitting, more (because of irritated fibers) or less (because of damaged or dead fibers) than normal fibers. A sudden trauma to a body part may crush pain nerves and result in acute—and, subsequently, chronic compressive— neuropathy. This in turn may cause chemical changes that cause inflammation, resulting in swelling, redness, and feelings of hotness. Examples of such disorders are painful diabetic neuropathy, post-herpetic neuralgia, and reflex sympathetic dystrophy. Medications and nerve blocks to help stabilize the nerve membranes are often used, as well as other pharmacotherapies, in attempting to manage this type of pain, which is often quite recalcitrant and becomes chronic in nature.

As Woessner (2003) noted, central pain is viewed as any pain that is the result of some dysfunction of neurons of the central nervous system (i.e., the brain and spinal cord). Examples of this are phantom limb pain and thalamic pain. These are especially difficult pain conditions to treat because the complex mechanisms involved are currently not well delineated. Treatment methods that directly affect neurons in the central nervous system must be used. Moreover, comprehensive interdisciplinary pain management programs, involving pharmacotherapy, psychosocial interventions, physical therapy, interventional techniques, and transcranial and body stimulation methods, are often necessary for treating these patients.

Treatment–Patient Matching

In subsequent chapters, I discuss pain management techniques, ranging from conservative nonoperative care, to palliative care, to more invasive techniques. As I emphasized in chapter 1, pain, especially when it becomes chronic in nature, often cannot be cured but only *managed*. This is also true for other chronic medical conditions, such as hypertension, diabetes, asthma, and so on. Moreover, as I discussed in chapter 1, there is good reason to move away from the traditional view of homogeneous pain patients. To be effective, treatments need to be matched to individual patients. As Borrie (2001) noted, psychologically based pain management can provide substantial relief for patients. He argued that this is because three of the four major components of pain (physical cause, muscle tension, attention, and interpretation) are primarily psychological in nature. Muscle tension, attentional focus, and interpretation are all responsive to psychologically based strategies (Turk & Gatchel, 2002). Thus, these components need to be considered in future treatment-matching attempts. The real task for a pain management specialist is to delineate the most important components that need the greatest attention for a particular patient. For example, one patient may have a great deal of muscle tension and anxiety associated with the pain. In this case, a program that provides a heavier dose of stress-reduction methods—such as relaxation training, biofeedback, and systematic desensitization—may be required. Another patient may have more interpretive problems as to what the pain means. This, in turn, may lead to greater catastrophizing and rumination problems. Providing a heavier dose of coping skills training and basic education may be important for this type of patient. The point is that every patient should be assessed as potentially having unique characteristics related to pain. It is up to the health care professional to evaluate what those characteristics are and then to tailor the treatment to best manage them. Of course, all of this should be accomplished in the context of an interdisciplinary program. Just because a patient may have some psychosocial issues that need to be addressed does not mean that biological aspects can be ignored. They all must be dealt with simultaneously, in an integrated manner.

Other Current Shortcomings in Managing Patients With Pain

Patients who pursue medical care for the high prevalence of common pain problems usually seek their primary-care physicians for advice (American Academy of Family Physicians, 1987). However, many times these pain problems are usually not associated with objective anatomical findings, and therefore a primary-care provider is challenged with the significant task of trying to evaluate and plan treatment for only a symptom. Moreover, often the symptoms presented are usually episodic and variable in terms of severity and the time since onset. An easy solution, such as splinting a broken arm or suturing an open cut, is usually not available. Because of a lack of training in understanding how to deal with pain, especially when it becomes chronic (where the role of patients' attitudes, beliefs, coping abilities, and other psychosocial factors, reviewed earlier, are important in the management and outcome), primary-care providers are significantly challenged with complex biopsychosocial problems for which they have been ill prepared to handle.

There have been a number of examples of how primary-care providers display a less-than-optimal approach in dealing with one type of pain: back pain. Such inadequacies have been observed in audiotaped analyses of the content and organization of primary-care visits for back pain (Turner, LeResche, Von Korff, & Ehrlich, 1998; Von Korff, 1999). In these analyses, it was found that the visits were quite similar. There was a brief social greeting, followed by a brief history of the problem and then a physical examination. Treatment recommendations were then made, usually consisting of prescription of medicine for acute pain and some advice about self-care. Thus, in general, these visits for back pain revolved around simple discussions about pain history, diagnosis, and possible medications. It was found that advice concerning patient self-management was very unfocused. Moreover, results of these studies revealed the following:

- Patient worries about the pain symptoms were really not asked about or addressed.
- Relatedly, patients often worried about serious disease or disability concerning the pain symptoms, without being told what the red flags or risks for these were.
- The physicians rarely took the opportunity to explain what was being looked for or ruled out during their evaluations.
- Staying active was many times recommended to some patients, without addressing how to do so safely.
- Physicians rarely spent time identifying functional difficulties that may be associated with the pain syndromes, or goals and plans for overcoming such difficulties.
- Relatedly, physicians did not attempt to identify and address such difficulties associated with performing work activities.
- Although many patients were already performing self-care activities, physicians missed opportunities to focus the visit on reinforcing such self-care but rather, focused on simply the medical management of pain.
- Diagnostic information provided to patients was often quite ambiguous, leaving patients uncertain about what improvement meant or when it could be expected.
- Current information about the natural progression of back pain was usually not provided, and many patients were simply given overly optimistic prognoses.
- Palliative care—typically, the prescription of nonsteroid anti-inflammatory medicines, elementary advice about exercise, and a possible referral to physical therapy—was usually prescribed. On a less frequent basis, opioids or muscle relaxants were prescribed.
- Rarely were the recommendations written down or were patients given any documentation of the recommendations.

The above findings prompted the investigators of these studies to suggest that there is an urgent need for improvements in physicians' behavior during these important aspects of the initial primary-care visit. This need for improvement is evidenced by the fact that approximately 30% of patients seeing a primary-care physician for back pain subsequently have persistent problems 12 months later, and approximately 20% of these patients continue to experience moderate or severe activity limitations due to back problems (Von Korff & Saunders, 1996). This is unfortunate, because there are some very effective evidence-based guidelines for the management of acute low back pain in primary care (McGuirk, King, Govind, Lowry, & Bogduk, 2001).

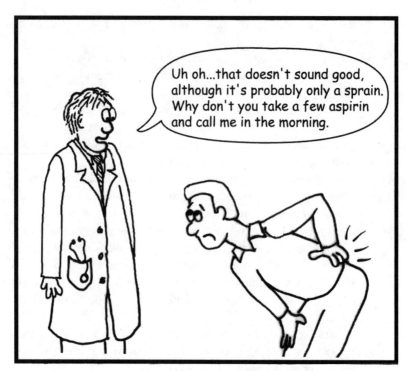

The approach that should not be taken when dealing with an acute pain episode patient.

As Pruitt and Von Korff (2002) highlighted, the insufficient preparation in medical school for dealing with pain problems, combined with time-pressured office visits in which complex biopsychosocial factors are present, as well as unrealistic patient expectations for immediate improvement, result in back problems being the most disliked condition seen by primary-care physicians. There obviously is a great need to rectify these multiple hindrances to quality back care and pain in general. A restructuring of the primary-care team and the services provided needs to be accomplished as a first line of defense for more effective pain management. Methods to assure the most effective management for primary-, secondary-, and tertiary-care settings are further reviewed in subsequent chapters of this book.

SUMMARY

Today, the biopsychosocial approach to pain assessment and management is the most widely embraced model in both the clinical and research arenas. It appropriately conceptualizes pain as a complex and dynamic interaction among physiological, psychological, and social factors that often results in, or at least maintains, pain. Because of the comprehensive nature of this model, one must be certain to assess and account for important interactions. For example, it is very important to become aware of the vagaries and difficulties inherent in differentiating among the constructs of pain, disability, and impairment. There is frequently a discordance among these constructs that creates potential problems for assessment and treatment personnel in selecting the best goal for developing a therapeutic plan and indexing therapeutic progress. Complicating this issue even more is the fact that there are three broad categories of measures—physical, psychological, and overt behavior/function—that have all been used to assess patients. These three major measurement categories, again, may not always display high concordance with one another. Fortunately, a number of recent works provide a comprehensive review of the best measurements of pain. In this chapter, I reviewed a number of commonly used biopsychosocial methods for evaluating the various constructs. Such evaluation is essential before developing a pain management strategy. I have emphasized that pain, especially when it becomes chronic in nature, often cannot be cured but only managed. Moreover, to be effective, such pain management procedures need to be matched to individual patients. A major task for a pain management specialist is to delineate the most important components needing the greatest attention for a particular patient. It is unfortunate that primary-care providers often display a less-than-optimal approach to dealing with pain. An example of this was provided in terms of back pain; however, the findings can be generalized to pain in general. The need is now greater than ever to conscientiously train health care professionals of all types in the most appropriate assessment and management techniques now available. Before this can be done, though, a better understanding of the various different ways pain can be classified needs to be discussed. This is the topic of the next chapter.

REFERENCES

American Academy of Family Physicians. (1987). *Facts about: Family practice*. Kansas City, MO: Author.

American Medical Association. (1993). *Guides to the evaluation of permanent impairment* (4th ed.). Chicago: Author.

American Psychiatric Association. (1994). *Diagnostic and statistical manual of mental disorders* (4th ed.). Washington, DC: Author.

Anderrson, G. B. J., Pope, M. H., Frymoyer, J. W., & Snook, S. H. (1991). Occupational low back pain: Assessment, treatment, and prevention. In M. H. Pope, G. B. J. Anderrson, J. W. Frymoyer, & D. B. Chaffin (Eds.), *Epidemiology and cost* (pp. 123–151). St. Louis, MO: Mosby Year Book.

Borrie, R. A. (2001, September–October). Thinking about pain: Psychologically based pain management can provide relief for pain patients. *Practical Pain Management, 22–24.*

Cocchiarella, L., & Anderson, G. (Eds.). (2001). *Guides to the evaluation of permanent impairment* (5th ed.). Chicago: American Medical Association Press.

Commission on Accreditation of Rehabilitation Facilities. (2001). *CARF manual.* Tucson, AZ: Author.

Dembe, A. E. (2000). Pain, function, impairment and disability: Implications for workers' compensation and other disability insurance systems. In T. G. Mayer, R. J. Gatchel, & P. B. Polatin (Eds.), *Occupational musculoskeletal disorders: Function, outcomes and evidence* (pp. 563–576). Philadelphia: Lippincott Williams & Wilkins.

Dubos, R. (1978). Health and creative adaptation. *Human Nature, 1*(1), 74–82.

Gatchel, R. J. (1996). Psychological disorders and chronic pain: Cause and effect relationships. In R. J. Gatchel & D. C. Turk (Eds.), *Psychological approaches to pain management: A practitioner's handbook* (pp. 33–52). New York: Guilford Press.

Gatchel, R. J. (1999). Perspectives on pain: A historical overview. In R. J. Gatchel & D. C. Turk (Eds.), *Psychosocial factors in pain: Critical perspectives* (pp. 3–17). New York: Guilford Press.

Gatchel, R. J. (2000). How practitioners should evaluate personality to help manage patients with chronic pain. In R. J. Gatchel & J. N. Weisberg (Eds.), *Personality characteristics of patients with pain* (pp. 241–257). Washington, DC: American Psychological Association.

Gatchel, R. J. (2001). *A compendium of outcome instruments for assessment and research of spinal disorders.* LaGrange, IL: North American Spine Society.

Gatchel, R. J., & Weisberg, J. N. (2000). *Personality characteristics of patients with pain.* Washington, DC: American Psychological Association.

Jensen, M. P. (2003). Questionnaire validation: A brief guide for readers of the research literature. *Clinical Journal of Pain, 19,* 345–352.

Joint Commission on Accreditation of Healthcare Organizations. (2000). *Pain assessment and management: An organizational approach.* Oakbrook, IL: Author.

Liang, M. H., & Sturrock, R. D. (1995). Evaluation of musculoskeletal symptoms. In J. H. Klippel & P. A. Dieppe (Eds.), *Practical rheumatology.* St. Louis, MO: Mosby.

Matheson, L. N. (1995). Functional capacity evaluation. In S. L. Demeter, G. Andersson, & G. Smith (Eds.), *Disability evaluation* (pp. 20–46). St. Louis, MO: Mosby.

Matheson, L. N. (2001). California Functional Capacity Protocol (Cal-FCP). In R. J. Gatchel (Ed.), *Compendium of outcome instruments for assessment and research of spinal disorders* (pp. 20–26). LaGrange, IL: North American Spine Society.

Matheson, L. N., & Ogden, D. (1993). *Work tolerance screening.* Trabuco Canyon, CA: Rehabilitation Institute of Southern California.

McGuirk, B., King, W., Govind, J., Lowry, J., & Bogduk, N. (2001). Safety, efficacy, and cost-effectiveness of evidence-based guidelines for the management of acute low back pain in primary care. *Spine, 26,* 2615–2622.

Pruitt, S. D., & Von Korff, M. (2002). Improving the management of low back pain: A paradigm shift for primary care. In D. C. Turk & R. J. Gatchel (Eds.), *Psychological approaches to pain management: A practitioner's handbook* (2nd ed.). New York: Guilford Press.

Robinson, R. C. (2001). Disability evaluation in painful conditions. In D. C. Turk & R. Melzack (Eds.), *Handbook of pain assessment* (2nd ed., pp. 248–272). New York: Guilford Press.

Tukey, J. W. (1979). Methodology and the statistician's responsibility for both accuracy and relevance. *Journal of the American Statistical Association, 74,* 786–793.

Turk, D. C. (1999). Biopsychosocial perspective on chronic pain. In R. J. Gatchel & D. C. Turk (Eds.), *Psychological approaches to pain management: A practitioner's handbook* (pp. 3–32). New York: Guilford Press.

Turk, D. C., & Gatchel, R. J. (Eds.). (2002). *Psychological approaches to pain management: A practitioner's handbook* (2nd ed.). New York: Guilford Press.

Turk, D. C., & Melzack, R. (2001). *Handbook of pain assessment* (2nd ed.). New York: Guilford Press.

Turk, D. C., & Monarch, E. S. (2002). Biopsychosocial perspective on chronic pain. In D. C. Turk & R. J. Gatchel (Eds.), *Psychological approaches to pain management: A practitioner's handbook* (2nd ed., pp. 3–29). New York: Guilford Press.

Turner, J. A., LeResche, L., Von Korff, M., & Ehrlich, K. (1998). Back pain in primary care: Patient characteristics, content of initial visit, and short-term outcomes. *Spine, 23,* 463–469.

Von Korff, M. (1999). Pain management in primary care: An individualized stepped-care approach. In R. J. Gatchel & D. C. Turk (Eds.), *Psychosocial factors in pain: Critical perspectives* (pp. 360–373). New York: Guilford Press.

Von Korff, M., & Saunders, K. (1996). The course of back pain in primary care. *Spine, 21,* 2833–2837.

Waddell, G. (1987). A new clinical method for the treatment of low back pain. *Spine, 12,* 632–644.

Woessner, J. (2003, January/February). A conceptual model of pain: Treatment modalities. *Practical Pain Management,* 26–36.

World Health Organization. (1980). *International classification of impairments, disabilities and handicaps.* Geneva, Switzerland: Author.

World Health Organization. (1989). *International statistical classification of diseases and related health problems.* Geneva, Switzerland: Author.

APPENDIX 2.1

Recommended Readings

Dembe, A. E. (2000). Pain, function, impairment and disability: Implications for workers' compensation and other disability insurance systems. In T. G. Mayer, R. J. Gatchel, & P. B. Polatin (Eds.), *Occupational musculoskeletal disorders: Function, outcomes and evidence* (pp. 563–576). Philadelphia: Lippincott Williams & Wilkins.

Jensen, M. P. (2003). Questionnaire validation: A brief guide for readers of the research literature. *Clinical Journal of Pain, 19,* 345–352.

Turk, D. C., & Gatchel, R. J. (Eds.). (2002). *Psychological approaches to pain management: A practitioner's handbook* (2nd ed.). New York: Guilford Press.

Turk, D. C., & Melzack, R. (2001). *Handbook of pain assessment* (2nd ed.). New York: Guilford Press.

Woessner, J. (2003, January–February). A conceptual model of pain: Treatment modalities. *Practical Pain Management,* 26–36.

3

ACUTE, CHRONIC, AND RECURRENT PAIN MANAGEMENT

One common way to classify pain is to consider it along a continuum of duration. Thus, pain . . . that is of relatively brief duration . . . is frequently referred to as acute pain. . . . Pain that persists for extended periods of time . . . is referred to as chronic pain. This duration continuum is inadequate, as it does not include acute recurrent pain.
—Turk and Melzack (2001)

There are various ways that pain can be classified. These can include the following:

- by the disease state causing pain as a symptom (e.g., pain associated with rheumatoid arthritis, pain associated with diabetic neuropathy, pain associated with cancer);
- by mechanism, in which pain is considered a symptom of a condition or disease, rather than merely a symptom (e.g., nociceptive; neuropathic); and
- by temporal profile (e.g., acute, chronic, episodic, or recurrent).

The temporal profile classification is most commonly used. This broad classification of pain duration is often used to better understand the biopsychosocial aspects that may be important when conducting assessment and treatment. For example, many times chronic pain is a result of unresolved acute pain episodes, resulting in accumulative biopsychosocial effects such as prolonged physical deconditioning, anxiety, and stress. It is obvious that this type of time categorization information can be extremely helpful in directing specific treatment approaches to the type of pain that is being evaluated (Gatchel & Oordt, 2003). *Acute pain* is usually indicative of tissue damage and is characterized by momentary intense noxious sensations (i.e., nociception). It serves as an important biological signal of potential tissue/ physical harm. Some anxiety may initially be precipitated, but prolonged physical and emotional distress usually is not. Indeed, anxiety, if mild, can be quite adaptive in that it stimulates behaviors needed for recovery, such as the seeking of medical attention, rest, and removal from the potentially harmful situation. As the nociception decreases, acute pain usually subsides.

Unlike acute pain, *chronic pain* persists. Chronic pain is traditionally defined as pain that lasts 6 months or longer, well past the normal healing period one would expect for its protective biological function. Arthritis, back injuries, and cancer can produce chronic-pain syndromes and, as the pain persists, it is often accompanied by emotional distress, such as depression, anger, and frustration. Such pain can also often significantly interfere with activities of daily living. There is much more health care utilization in an attempt to find some relief from the pain symptoms, and the pain has a tendency to become a preoccupation of an individual's everyday living. As I discuss later in this chapter, as pain becomes more chronic in nature, there is an increased likelihood of greater psychosocial distress sequelae.

Intense, *episodic pain*, recurring for more than 3 months, is often referred to as *recurrent pain*. Recurrent pain episodes are usually brief (as are acute pain episodes); however, the recurring nature of this type of pain makes it similar to chronic pain in that it is very distressing to patients. Such episodes may develop without a well-defined cause and then may begin to generate an array of emotional reactions, such as anxiety, stress, and depression and feelings of helplessness. Often, pain medication is used to control the intensity of the recurrent pain, but it is not usually helpful in reducing the frequency of the episodes that a person experiences. It should also be noted that patients often find it difficult to distinguish between chronic and recurrent pain. Patients will frequently present with "chronic-like" symptoms from prolonged episodes of, say, headache or back pain. These do not always fit the description of chronic pain but are usually persistent and can be as disabling. It should be kept in mind that all pain, be it acute, chronic, or recurrent, may often be accompanied by emotional distress. A health care professional will need to understand the different factors, such as psychological, sociocultural, environmental, and pathophysiological (i.e., a comprehensive biopsychosocial evaluation) associated with all three types of pain in order to treat such pain and predict patients' responses to treatment.

A CONCEPTUAL MODEL OF HOW ACUTE PAIN DEVELOPS INTO CHRONIC PAIN

Before I discuss pain management options, it is worthwhile to develop a conceptualization of how acute pain can progress into a chronic-pain situation. I (Gatchel, 1991, 1996) have characterized this progression from acute to chronic pain as a three-stage model (see Figure 3.1). In Stage 1 of

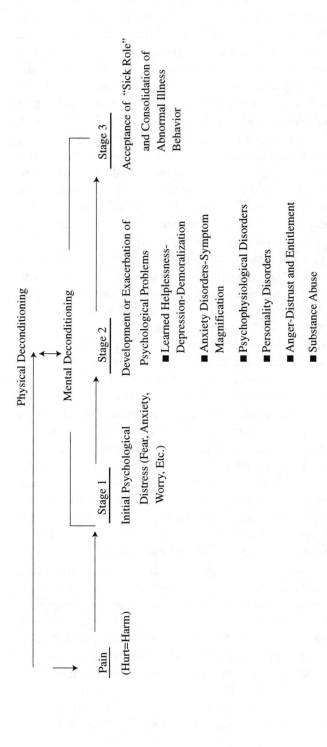

Figure 3.1. Gatchel's three-stage model. From "Early Development of Physical and Mental Deconditioning in Painful Spinal Disorders," by R. J. Gatchel, in *Contemporary Conservative Care for Painful Spinal Disorders*, p. 282, edited by T. G. Mayer, V. Mooney, and R. J. Gatchel, 1991, Philadelphia: Lea & Febiger. Copyright 1991 by Lea & Febiger. Reprinted with permission.

this model, referred to as the *acute phase*, normal emotional reactions (such as fear, anxiety, and worry) develop subsequent to the patient's perception of pain. As noted above, this is a natural emotional reaction that often serves a protective function by prompting the individual to heed the pain signal and, if necessary, seek medical attention for it. However, if the perception of pain exists beyond a 2- to 4-month period (which is usually considered a normal healing time for most pain syndromes), the pain begins to develop into a more chronic condition, leading into Stage 2 of the model. During this second stage, psychological and behavioral problems are often exacerbated. Learned helplessness, anger, distress, and somatization are typical symptoms of patients in Stage 2. Often, the extent of these symptoms usually depends on the individual's preexisting personality and psychosocial structure, in addition to socioeconomic and environmental conditions. For example, depressive symptoms are greatly exacerbated during this stage for an individual with a premorbid depressive personality who is seriously affected economically by loss of a job due to the pain and disability. Similarly, an individual who had premorbid hypochondriacal characteristics and who receives a great deal of secondary gain (e.g., sympathy from others) from remaining disabled will most likely display a great deal of somatization and symptom magnification.

The model proposes a *diathesis–stress* perspective, in which the stress of coping with pain can lead to exacerbation of the individual's underlying psychological characteristics. This model proposes not that there is a preexisting pain-prone personality; but rather that patients bring with them certain predisposing personality and psychological characteristics (i.e., they have a *diathesis*) that is then exacerbated by the *stress* of attempting to cope with the now-chronic nature of the pain. Indeed, the relationship between stress and the exacerbation of mental health problems has been documented in the scientific literature (Barrett, Rose, & Klerman, 1979). This is not to say that predisposing factors make chronic pain a psychogenic disorder and that it is all in the person's head. Again, the chronic problem represents a complex interaction between physical factors and psychosocioeconomic variables.

Finally, the progression to complex interactions of physical, psychological, and social processes characterize Stage 3, which represents the chronic phase of the model. As the result of the chronic nature of the pain experience, and the stress that it creates, the patient's life begins to revolve around the pain and the behaviors that maintain it. The patient begins to adopt a "sick role," in which any excuse from social and occupational responsibilities becomes routine. As a consequence, the patient now becomes accustomed to the avoidance of responsibility, and other reinforcers maintain such maladaptive behavior.

Superimposed on these three stages is what is referred to as the *physical deconditioning syndrome*, originally delineated by Mayer and Gatchel (1988).

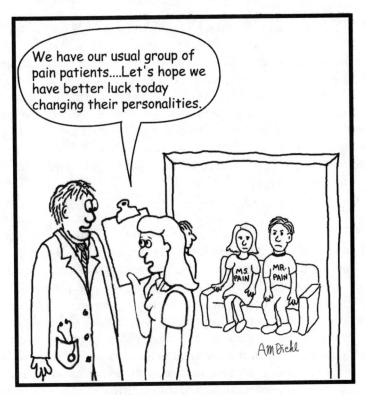

The "pain-prone personality" myth.

This is a significant decrease in physical capacity (such as strength, mobility, and endurance) resulting from disuse and the resultant atrophy of the injured area. There is usually a two-way pathway between the physical deconditioning and the three stages described above. For example, physical deconditioning can feed back and negatively affect the emotional well-being and self-esteem of individuals. This can lead to further negative psychosocial sequelae. Conversely, negative emotional reactions, such as depression, can feed back to physical functioning (e.g., by decreasing the motivation to get involved in work or recreational activities and thereby contributing further to physical deconditioning).

Of course, the key in treating pain is to not let it progress to the chronic stage, where more complex biopsychosocial problems develop. Good patient care, which usually involves merely taking steps to reassure the patient that the pain is only temporary (thus allaying a great deal of the patient's anxiety and fears), and appropriate medication management if required, goes a long way to help prevent the patient from becoming overly preoccupied with the pain and helps to prevent premature catastrophizing about the symptoms.

PRIMARY, SECONDARY, AND TERTIARY PAIN MANAGEMENT

Distinctions among primary, secondary, and tertiary pain management care, highlighted earlier in the clinical research by Mayer et al. (1995), and subsequently reviewed by me (Gatchel, 1996), are helpful because they suggest that the type of biopsychosocial treatment required for each is substantially different. In discussing back pain rehabilitation, for example, *primary care* is applied usually to acute cases of pain of limited severity. Basic symptom-control methods are used in relieving pain during the normal early healing period. Frequently, some basic psychological reassurance that the acute pain episode is temporary, and will soon be resolved, is quite effective. *Secondary care* represents "reactivation" treatment administered to patients who do not improve simply through the normal healing process. It is administered during the transition from acute (primary) care to the patient's eventual return to work. Such treatment has been designed to promote a return to productivity before advanced physical deconditioning and significant psychosocial barriers to returning to work occur. At this phase, more active psychosocial intervention may need to be administered to patients who do not appear to be progressing. Finally, *tertiary care* requires an interdisciplinary and intensive treatment approach. It is intended for patients suffering the effects of physical deconditioning and chronic disability. In general, it differs from secondary care in regard to the intensity of rehabilitation services required, including psychosocial and disability management. The critical elements of interdisciplinary care, such as functional restoration (Mayer & Gatchel, 1988), involve the following:

- formal, repeated quantification of physical deficits to guide, individualize, and monitor physical training progress;
- psychosocial and socioeconomic assessment to guide, individualize, and monitor disability behavior-oriented interventions and outcomes;
- a multimodal disability management program using cognitive–behavioral approaches;
- psychopharmacological interventions for detoxification and psychological management;
- an interdisciplinary, medically directed team approach with formal staffing, frequent team conferences, and low staff-to-patient ratios; and
- ongoing outcome assessment using standardized objective criteria.

Such interdisciplinary biopsychosocial treatment programs have been shown to be extremely efficacious, as well as cost effective, in successfully managing chronic-pain patients, relative to less intensive, single-modality treatment programs (e.g., Deschner & Polatin, 2000; Mayer & Polatin, 2000).

In terms of primary and secondary care, the clinician must be aware of many psychosocial factors that can contribute to an acute pain episode becoming subacute and then chronic. A patient may progress through a number of stages (reviewed earlier in this chapter) as his or her pain and disability become more chronic (i.e., Stages 2 and 3). These may create significant barriers to recovery if they are not effectively dealt with. These barriers to recovery include the psychosocial variables discussed earlier, as well as functional, legal, and work-related issues that can greatly interfere with the patient's return to full functioning and a productive lifestyle. Treatment personnel must also be alert to potential secondary gains of continued disability (which I discuss more fully in chap. 7). It is important that members of the health care team be knowledgeable about all psychosocial issues while the patient is in treatment. This knowledge allows staff members not only to understand and serve the patient better but also to be more effective in problem solving if the patient's physical progress is slow or nonexistent. At other times, real interfering circumstances (e.g., transportation problems, child care) may be used as "smoke screens" or excuses for suboptimal performance and failure to adhere to the treatment regimen. Indeed, failure to make physical progress generally indicates psychosocial barriers to recovery. These barriers to recovery issues must be effectively assessed and brought to the attention of the entire treatment team. Steps can then be taken to understand their origins and avoid their interference with treatment goals.

In the next chapter, I discuss a *stepwise approach* to pain evaluation. Also, in chapter 5 I review a *three-step care framework* that is similar to the primary, secondary, and tertiary pain management distinctions described above. Step 1 is the lowest intensity of intervention, which consists of addressing a patient's fear and avoidance belief about pain through education, information, and advice about the importance of returning to activities of daily living as soon as possible. Step 2 refers to the need for increasing intensity of intervention and is reserved for patients who may continue to report pain 6 to 8 weeks following the onset of an episode and who demonstrate persistent limitations in activities of daily living. Finally, Step 3 is for those patients who fail to improve with either Step 1 or Step 2 interventions. These patients continue to experience significant disability and are at risk for becoming permanently disabled. Intervention at this step may be much more costly and complex than Step 1 and Step 2 interventions. It is at this step where more complex biopsychosocial issues need to be addressed, using an intensive interdisciplinary treatment approach.

ACUTE PAIN MANAGEMENT

The role of a psychologist is often less vital in the management of acute pain than it is in the management of more chronic or persistent pain, in part because there is a wide variety of pharmacological agents capable of bringing about rapid relief for many acute pain conditions. However, as Williams (1996) noted, psychologists have identified additional effective methods of acute pain assessment, and have highlighted to medical colleagues the other important biopsychosocial factors, including:

- the role of behavioral and emotional modulation of acute pain,
- the important role of beliefs in the perception of pain,
- the beneficial effects of brief coping skills in managing acute pain,
- the frequent need for brief pharmacological methods of managing acute pain, and
- cognitive factors that can impede adequate pain control.

The underreporting of acute pain can often lead to needless pain escalation, as well as accompanying physical complications. This underreporting is not an isolated problem. Even though the single best measure of pain is the patient's own self-report, how such a self-report is obtained varies greatly from one practice to the next. For example, Price, Bush, Long, and Harkins (1994) evaluated 218 independent physicians concerning their preferences of obtaining measurements and found the following: Fifty-six percent preferred numerical rating scales, 19.5% preferred verbal rating scales, and only 7% preferred visual analog scales. *Numerical rating scales* request patients to rate the intensity of their pain in terms of a numerical descriptor (e.g., 0–10), with the endpoints usually having verbal descriptors such as *no pain* and *worse pain*. One disadvantage of this type of rating is the inability of some patients, especially older adults and members of different cultural groups, to actually conceptualize pain (and actual bodily sensation) as a specific number. A *verbal rating scale* requests patients to use one word from a list of adjectives to rate their pain intensity. These adjectives are subsequently transformed into a standardized pain intensity score. Thus, for example, a 12-point item adjective checklist may be administered, with adjectives varying from *not noticeable*, to *moderate*, all the way to *excruciating*. A drawback of this type of scale is that it is often difficult for both the patient and clinician to remember all of the adjectives, thus possibly affecting test–retest reliability and attempts to monitor change. Moreover, it is often observed that patients have a tendency to use the middle adjectives more frequently than the endpoints, thus limiting the range of responses.

Finally, a *visual analog scale* is a straight line (usually 10 centimeters long) with verbal descriptors at the endpoints, such as *no pain* at one end and *excruciating pain* at the other (Jensen & Karoly, 2001). The patient is simply requested to place a mark on the line to indicate the intensity of his or her pain. A ruler is usually then used to measure the length of the line where the mark is made. Visual analog scales have many advantages because they are visual in nature, and they allow patients to mark anywhere along the line without potential descriptors negatively influencing their responses.

The Joint Commission on Accreditation of Health Care Organizations now requires that pain severity (because it is the *fifth vital sign*) be documented using a pain scale, such as one of the scales described above. One that may be easily used was presented in chapter 1 (Exhibit 1.1). In addition, the patient's own words describing his or her pain, pain location, duration, aggravating and alleviating factors, present pain management regimens and effectiveness, effects of pain, the patient's pain goal, as well as the physical examination, all should be documented at the initial assessment. This initiative has created a new mandate to successfully assess pain and should lead to more consistent approaches from one clinician to the next. Williams (1996) reviewed the importance of a number of important issues when treating acute pain patients, as listed below.

- Many patients prefer playing an active role in their medical treatment. In such instances, these patients can be trained in active pain management techniques such as relaxation or distraction techniques.
- There are certain cognitive factors that may impede adequate pain control. Factors such as incorrect beliefs about the meaning of pain and its expected duration can be addressed by providing patients with appropriate information and communication about such issues. Appropriate compliance with any prescribed treatment is also important to monitor.
- Often, involving family members and significant others in the pain assessment–treatment process is important because of the beneficial effects that social support can have on medical conditions of all types, including pain. An overview of a family-focused session that I have developed for my program is presented in Appendix 3.2. This session is usually conducted near the end of treatment, when all the issues reviewed have been addressed with the patient (these issues are discussed in the chapters that follow).

Finally, if acute pain is appropriately dealt with at the primary-care setting, there is definitely the significant potential to reduce the chances of chronicity, as well as to minimize disability and limit excessive use of health care services (Malmivaara et al., 1995). The major approaches that should be diligently adhered to in the primary-care setting when treating patients reporting pain, as summarized by Gatchel and Oordt (2003), are the following:

- Discuss the rationale for the physical examination as well as any diagnostic tests that are needed.
- Assess the patient's pain (using the Joint Commission on Accreditation of Health Care Organizations guidelines), especially the pain's interference with daily activity.
- Reassure common patient worries regarding the source and meaning of pain, possible future disability or activity limitations, and so on.
- Relate realistic and reassuring prognostic statements.
- Encourage self-care activities, such as exercise, continuation of routine activities, and medication management when appropriate. Offer praise or support for such efforts.
- Address patients' coping abilities, attitudes, beliefs, and daily behaviors related to the pain.
- Collaborate with patients to determine whether they can reliably adhere to treatment recommendations.
- Provide information and education about pain, preferably in a written booklet format.
- Write down the treatment recommendation for each patient.
- Follow up with patients after the initial visit to evaluate treatment gains.

EPISODIC OR RECURRENT PAIN MANAGEMENT

The management of headache disorders is a good example of how episodic or recurrent pain disorders can be effectively dealt with. Lipchik, Holroyd, and Nash (2002) provided a comprehensive review of clinical developments in the management of recurrent-headache disorders that have occurred during the last 25 years. Recurrent headaches are one of the most common, yet least understood, physical problems today. Overall, the prevalence of all types of headache is well over 60% of the population; this accounts for approximately 18.3 million outpatient medical visits per year (Gauthier, Ivers, & Carrier, 1996). Headaches can occur in isolation or as part of another medical disease, or they can signify the onset of something more severe, such as a brain tumor or a subarachnoid hemorrhage (Lance, 2000). When a headache occurs repeatedly, and is not determined to be a symptom of another type of medical disorder, it is collectively referred to as a *benign idiopathic headache*. A classification system developed by the

International Headache Society (Ollsen, 1988) proposes that headaches can initially be divided into primary or secondary disorders. Primary disorders are equivalent to benign, idiopathic headache disorders, whereas secondary headache disorders are the result of a side effect of some other medical disorder. Within the primary headache disorder classification, moreover, four specific categories are recognized: (a) migraine, (b) tension-type, (c) cluster, and (d) miscellaneous headaches. These headaches may be considered episodic if they occur fewer than 15 days in the month and considered chronic if they occur more often. It should also be noted that a subset of chronic headaches can also be associated with overuse of acute-headache medications.

Of course, before any pain management program is initiated with headache sufferers, a thorough biopsychosocial assessment needs to be conducted to rule out the headache as secondary to a disease state or structural abnormality, as well as to gather a comprehensive headache history and diagnostic data to determine what type of headache it is. Indeed, a complete medical evaluation is a necessity before any patient with pain is treated. The evaluation of possible comorbid psychiatric disorders; the degree of anxiety and depression; the impact of the headache on work, family, and social functioning; antecedents of headache onset; and information on the patient's medication regimen history should also all be systematically collected. It is also worthwhile to have patients keep a headache diary to provide information concerning headache onset, what activities were engaged in on onset, ratings of pain intensity and duration, and any medication used. For compliance purposes, it is usually best to request this information four times a day: (a) when arising in the morning, (b) at lunch time, (c) at dinner time, and (d) at bedtime. Not only do such diaries provide important assessment information before the start of treatment for baseline purposes, but also their continuation throughout treatment will provide a barometer of treatment progression and ultimate clinical effectiveness. Exhibit 3.1A provides an example of a basic headache diary, and Exhibit 3.1B presents a more general diary. Of course, such diaries may be used for other types of pain.

Lipchik et al. (2002) noted that a variety of qualitative and analytic reviews strongly indicate that cognitive–behavioral treatment yields a 40% to 60% reduction in migraine or tension-type headaches in adults. Moreover, the Agency for Health Care Research and Quality (Goslin, Gray, & McCrory, 2001) has indicated that it is an empirically supported treatment in clinical practice for the management of migraine headaches when the treatment includes the following: relaxation training, thermal biofeedback combined with relaxation training, EMG biofeedback, and cognitive–behavioral therapy. Lipchik et al. went on to list the major components that should be used in pain management programs for recurrent pain disorders

EXHIBIT 3.1A
Headache Diary

Name	Date

Time of Headache _____

Intensity of Headache
(1 = very mild . . . 10 = very intense) _____

What were you doing at time of
  headache onset? _____

Duration of Headache _____

Medications Taken _____

Time of Last Meal Before Headache _____

Hours of Sleep Night Before Headache _____

<u>GENERAL COMMENTS</u>

such as headache (see Appendix 3.3). Many of these components can be used for other types of pain as well. Note that relaxation training is an important component of this, as well as most other, pain management programs. Some general relaxation training protocols that can be used are presented in Appendix 3.4. These are modified adaptations from some of those presented by Fuller (1984). Likewise, general instructions for biofeedback can be found in Appendix 3.5. Biofeedback therapy should be initiated

EXHIBIT 3.1B
Daily Pain Log

NAME: _____   0 = None . . . 10 = Extreme

	Pain	General	Remarks
DATE:			
Morning			
Noon			
After Work/Before Dinner			
Before Bed			
DATE:			
Morning			
Noon			
After Work/Before Dinner			
Before Bed			
DATE:			
Morning			
Noon			
After Work/Before Dinner			
Before Bed			
DATE:			
Morning			
Noon			
After Work/Before Dinner			
Before Bed			

only after appropriate relaxation training, because the latter skills will facilitate the biofeedback learning process.

Using a technique such as that presented in Appendix 3.3, which is referred to as *minimal-therapist-contact treatment*, Lipchik et al. (2002) emphasized that such a format can reduce the cost and increase the availability of such treatment in medical settings, as well as reduce barriers to the integration of biopsychosocial treatments into the medical setting.

CHRONIC PAIN MANAGEMENT

The most prevalent chronic pain conditions include the following:

- pain related to irritable bowel syndrome (20%),
- osteoarthritis (15%),
- low back pain (14%),
- chronic pelvic pain (12%),

- migraine headaches (12%),
- chronic tension headaches (3%), and
- fibromyalgia (2%).

As I noted earlier in this chapter, when pain becomes chronic, a more intensive tertiary care or interdisciplinary treatment approach is required because of the significant effects of physical deconditioning and chronic disability. The critical elements of this interdisciplinary approach are reviewed below. A number of reviews have documented the clinical effectiveness of such interdisciplinary treatment of chronic-pain patients (e.g., Deschner & Polatin, 2000; Gatchel, 1999; Okifuji, 2003; Wright & Gatchel, 2002). Such interdisciplinary programs are needed for chronic-pain patients who have complex needs and requirements. Although they represent a small minority of pain patients, there nevertheless is a significant number of patients who have failed to benefit from the combination of spontaneous healing and short-term, symptom-focused treatment. They have also become financial burdens on their insurance carriers as well as the health care system in general. They have often failed to experience significant pain relief after repeated and extended contacts with several different physicians and other health care providers. Psychosocial distress, physical deconditioning, secondary gains and losses, and medication issues often complicate their presentation. Therefore, this stage of treatment is much more complex and demanding of health care professionals. As such, the strengths of multiple disciplines working together to address the complex issues confronting chronic-pain patients are greatly needed. The overall therapeutic focus should be toward independence and autonomy while acknowledging when certain physical limitations cannot be overcome. The Commission on Accreditation of Rehabilitation Facilities requires that a certified pain management team include, at a minimum, a physician, specialized nurse, physical therapist, and clinical psychologist or psychiatrist. However, often an occupational therapist is required because return-to-work and vocational retraining issues become important in managing chronic-pain patients.

Finally, one variant of interdisciplinary chronic pain management programs—functional restoration—was extensively reviewed by Mayer and Polatin (2000). The interdisciplinary treatment team consists of the following:

- The *physician* serves as a medical director of the treatment plan, and he or she must have a firm background in providing medical rehabilitation for the types of pain disorders frequently encountered. Formal training may vary from anesthesiology, orthopedic surgery, psychiatry, occupational medicine, to internal medicine. The physician needs to assume a direct role in the medical management of the patient's pain by providing the medical history to the treatment team and by taking direct responsibility for medication management for any other medical interventions. Often, other team members and outside consultants may be involved in the medical treatment of the patient, but it is the physician's responsibility to coordinate these medical contributions to the patient's care.

- Although not all programs use nursing services, any pain management program that provides anesthesiology services, involving injections, nerve blocks, and other medical procedures, will require a *nurse*. The nurse assists the physician, follows up the procedures, and may interact with patients in the role of case manager, as well as providing patient education. The nurse may be viewed as a physician-extender and educator who has a strong impact on the patient.

- Although the physician and nurse play a major role in managing the physical status of patients, the *psychologist* plays the leading role in the day-to-day maintenance of the psychosocial aspects and status of the patient's care. Significant psychosocial barriers to positive outcomes of the treatment may develop as a patient progresses from acute through subacute to the chronic stage of a pain syndrome (reviewed earlier in this chapter). The psychologist is responsible for performing a full psychosocial evaluation, which includes identification of psychosocial barriers to recovery and the assessment of the patient's psychological strengths and weaknesses. A cognitive–behavioral treatment approach can then be used to address important psychosocial issues, such as pain-related depression, anxiety, fear, as well as psychopathology. A cognitive–behavioral treatment approach has been found to be the most appropriate modality to use with patients in a program such as this.

- The *physical therapist* interacts daily with the patient regarding any issues regarding physical progression toward recovery. Effective communication with other team members is crucial so that the patient's fear of exercise will not interfere with his or her reconditioning effort. The physical therapist also helps to educate the patient by addressing the physiological bases of pain and teaching ways of reducing the severity of pain episodes through the use of appropriate body mechanics and pacing.

- The *occupational therapist* is involved in both physical and vocational aspects of the patient's treatment. The great majority of patients participating in an interdisciplinary program are likely to not be working because of their pain. Often, they have become pessimistic about the prospect of returning to work.

The occupational therapist addresses these vocational issues and the physical determinants of underlying disability. This therapist also plays an important educational role in teaching patients techniques for managing pain on the job in ways that do not jeopardize their employment status. Finally, the occupational therapist can play an important role as case manager in contacting employers to obtain job descriptions and other information, as well as vocational retraining if necessary.

- Constant, effective communication among all treatment personnel, during which patient progress can be discussed and evaluated, is required. This is important so patients hear the same treatment philosophy and message from each of the treatment team members. Indeed, many times patients are in conflict about their own future treatment and may seek out any conflict between team members and use it to compromise treatment goals.
- A formal interdisciplinary treatment team meeting should occur at least once a week to review patient progress and to make any modifications in the treatment plan for each patient. Individually tailoring treatment for patients is essential.
- Evaluating and monitoring treatment outcomes in a systematic fashion is essential not only for treatment outcome evaluations but also for quality-assurance purposes for the treatment team.

The clinical effectiveness of functional restoration has been well documented. Indeed, Gatchel and Turk (1999) and Turk (2002) have reviewed both the therapeutic and cost effectiveness of interdisciplinary programs, such as functional restoration, for the wide range of chronic pain conditions. Health care professionals fortunately now have in their treatment armamentarium the ability to effectively manage what used to be recalcitrant chronic-pain syndromes.

SUMMARY

Although there are various ways that pain can be classified, a temporal profile (e.g., acute, chronic, episodic, or recurrent) is most commonly used today. This allows a better understanding of the biopsychosocial aspects that may be important when conducting assessments and treatments. For example, chronic pain is the result of unresolved acute pain episodes, often resulting in accumulated biopsychosocial effects such as prolonged physical deconditioning and significant emotional distress. I have presented a conceptual model of how acute pain develops into chronic pain that further emphasizes the greater degree of negative psychosocial sequelae associated with chronic pain. As I have emphasized, the key in treating pain is not to let it progress to the chronic stage, where more such complex biopsychosocial problems develop. Relatedly, I presented a different type of pain management associated with this temporal profile classification: primary, secondary, and tertiary pain management. I also reviewed general assessment and treatment issues associated with these different categories of pain. In Part II of this book, I provide a more comprehensive evaluation of pain assessment and management techniques.

REFERENCES

Barrett, J. F., Rose, R. M., & Klerman, G. L. (Eds.). (1979). *Stress and mental disorder*. New York: Raven Press.

Deschner, M., & Polatin, P. B. (2000). Interdisciplinary programs: Chronic pain management. In T. G. Mayer, R. J. Gatchel, & P. B. Polatin (Eds.), *Occupational musculoskeletal disorders: Function, outcomes, and evidence* (pp. 629–637). Philadelphia: Lippincott, Williams & Wilkins.

Fuller, G. D. (1984). *Biofeedback: Methods and procedures in clinical practice*. San Francisco: Biofeedback Press.

Gatchel, R. J. (1991). Early development of physical and mental deconditioning in painful spinal disorders. In T. G. Mayer, V. Mooney, & R. J. Gatchel (Eds.), *Contemporary conservative care for painful spinal disorders* (pp. 278–289). Philadelphia: Lea & Febiger.

Gatchel, R. J. (1996). Psychological disorders and chronic pain: Cause and effect relationships. In R. J. Gatchel & D. C. Turk (Eds.), *Psychological approaches to pain management: A practitioner's handbook* (pp. 33–52). New York: Guilford Press.

Gatchel, R. J. (1999). Perspectives on pain: A historical overview. In R. J. Gatchel & D. C. Turk (Eds.), *Psychosocial factors in pain: Critical perspectives* (pp. 3–17). New York: Guilford Press.

Gatchel, R. J., & Oordt, M. S. (2003). *Clinical health psychology and primary care: Practical advice and clinical guidance for successful collaboration*. Washington, DC: American Psychological Association.

Gatchel, R. J., & Turk, D. C. (1999). Interdisciplinary treatment of chronic pain patients. In R. J. Gatchel & D. C. Turk (Eds.), *Psychosocial factors in pain: Critical perspectives* (pp. 435–444). New York: Guilford Press.

Gauthier, J. P., Ivers, H., & Carrier, S. (1996). Non-pharmacological approaches in the management of recurrent headache disorder and their comparison and combination with pharmacological therapy. *Clinical Psychology Review, 16*, 543–571.

Goslin, R., Gray, R., & McCrory, D. (2001). *Behavioral and physical treatment for migraine headache: Technical Review 2.2*. Retrieved May 15, 2001, from http://www.clinpol.mc.duke.edu

Jensen, M. P., & Karoly, P. (2001). Self-report scales and procedures for assessing pain in adults. In D. C. Turk & R. Melzack (Eds.), *Handbook of pain assessment* (2nd ed., pp. 15–34). New York: Guilford Press.

Lance, J. W. (2000). Headache and face pain. *Medical Journal of Australia, 172*, 450–455.

Lipchik, G. L., Holroyd, K. A., & Nash, J. M. (2002). Cognitive–behavior management of recurrent headache disorders: A minimal-therapist-contact approach. In D. C. Turk & R. J. Gatchel (Eds.), *Psychological approaches to pain management: A practitioner's handbook* (2nd ed., pp. 365–389). New York: Guilford Press.

Malmivaara, A., Hakkinen, U., Aro, T., Heinrichs, M. L., Koskenniemi, L., Kuosma, E., et al. (1995). The treatment of acute low back pain—bed rest, exercises, or ordinary activity? *New England Journal of Medicine, 332*, 351–355.

Mayer, T. G., & Gatchel, R. J. (1988). *Functional restoration for spinal disorders: The sports medicine approach.* Philadelphia: Lea & Febiger.

Mayer, T. G., & Polatin, P. B. (2000). Tertiary nonoperative interdisciplinary programs: The functional restoration variant of the outpatient chronic pain management program. In T. G. Mayer, R. J. Gatchel, & P. B. Polatin (Eds.), *Occupational musculoskeletal disorders: Function, outcomes, and evidence* (pp. 639–649). Philadelphia: Lippincott, Williams & Wilkins.

Mayer, T. G., Polatin, P., Smith, B., Smith, C., Gatchel, R., Herring, S. A., et al. (1995). Spine rehabilitation: Secondary and tertiary nonoperative care. *Spine, 20*, 2060–2066.

Okifuji, A. (2003). Interdisciplinary pain management with pain patients: Evidence for its effectiveness. *Seminars in Pain Management, 1*, 110–119.

Ollsen, J. C. (1988). Classification and diagnostic criteria for headache disorders, cranial neuralgias and facial pain: Headache Classification Committee of the International Headache Society. *Caphalalgia, 8*(Suppl. 7), 1–96.

Price, D. D., Bush, F. M., Long, S., & Harkins, S. W. (1994). A comparison of pain measurement characteristics of mechanical visual analogue and simple numerical rating scales. *Pain, 56*, 217–226.

Turk, D. C. (2002). Clinical effectiveness and cost effectiveness of treatment for patients with chronic pain. *Clinical Journal of Pain, 18*, 355–365.

Turk, D. C., & Melzack, P. (2001). *Handbook of pain assessment* (2nd ed.). New York: Guilford Press.

Williams, D. A. (1996). Acute pain management. In R. J. Gatchel & D. C. Turk (Eds.), *Psychological approaches to pain management: A practitioner's handbook* (pp. 55–77). New York: Guilford Press.

Wright, A. R., & Gatchel, R. J. (2002). Occupational musculoskeletal pain and disability. In D. C. Turk & R. J. Gatchel (Eds.), *Psychological approaches to pain management: A practitioner's handbook* (2nd ed., pp. 349–364). New York: Guilford Press.

APPENDIX 3.1

Recommended Readings

Gatchel, R. J., & Turk, D. C. (1999). Interdisciplinary treatment of chronic pain patients. In R. J. Gatchel & D. C. Turk (Eds.), *Psychosocial factors in pain: Critical perspectives* (pp. 435–444). New York: Guilford Press.

Okifuji, A. (2003). Interdisciplinary pain management with pain patients: Evidence for its effectiveness. *Seminars in Pain Management, 1,* 110–119.

Turk, D. C. (2002). Clinical effectiveness and cost effectiveness of treatment for patients with chronic pain. *Clinical Journal of Pain, 18,* 355–365.

Woessner, J. (2002, September/October). A conceptual model of pain. *Practical Pain Management, 2,* 8–16.

Worsham, S. L., & Ziegler, R. R. (2002, January/February). Multidisciplinary approaches to pain. *Practical Pain Management,* 16–20.

APPENDIX 3.2

A Family-Focused Session

1. Goals

The first part of this session will review some basic information about pain and what things affect it. We will discuss the relationship between pain and stress, as well as theories of pain as they relate to pain management. We will then talk about methods that can be used to cope with pain. You will also be provided with information on how you can help with this pain management process in order to decrease the pain and prevent it from recurring.

Gate-Control Theory of Pain

The gate-control model of pain describes how thoughts, feelings, and behavior affect pain. Pain is a subjective experience that varies between people and different situations.

- The pain message begins at the site of injury, then a signal of pain is transmitted to the brain, and an individual becomes aware of the pain sensation.
- A gate located in your brain determines your perception of pain. This gate can be opened or closed, which determines the amount of pain you feel. Coping strategies can close the gate, increase your ability to cope, and give you more control over your pain.
- Thoughts that open the gate are focusing on the pain, negative thinking, and nonconstructive thinking. Feelings that open

the gate are feelings of stress, tension, sadness, hopelessness, helplessness, and anger.

- Many people experience these feelings at some point in time, and it is a normal reaction when experiencing prolonged pain. But it is important to identify your negative, self-defeating thoughts and feelings to ensure that you don't stay focused on them.
- Behaviors that can open the gate may be poor nutrition, inactivity, inadequate sleep, smoking, or lack of exercise. These factors predispose a person to pain, increasing his or her vulnerability to pain and to more intense pain.

2. Pain–Stress Cycle

Stress and tension can interfere with one's ability to control pain and can keep one from enjoying things that one normally would. Stress and tension can cause fatigue and increased pain.

- They are normal reactions that evolved from our natural fight-or-flight response, which occurs when a situation is perceived as threatening.
- A certain level of tension is needed to function effectively, but often our tension level exceeds this.
- Scientific and clinical studies have demonstrated that relaxation is effective in the management of pain. We teach relaxation in this program!
- The pain–stress cycle plays a key role in understanding how your feelings and behaviors affect pain.
- Interventions at any point in the cycle affect other parts of the cycle. If pain is lowered, then stress and worry decrease. If stress and worry are lowered, then pain is decreased.
- Pain, stress, and worry are related, and a change in one affects the others. Stress, tension, or worry can increase pain intensity and decrease a person's pain threshold.
- Many people who have persistent pain find themselves stuck in a cycle of feeling stress, increasing tension, and pain. In understanding how your behaviors are contributing to your stress/tension–pain cycle, you can gain more control over your pain.

3. Negative Thinking and Pain

People with chronic pain often have a number of negative thoughts and see the world through a type of negative filter. Patients in our program learn to identify and change negative thoughts that may be causing unnecessary stress, tension, and pain in their lives. There is a direct connection between how you *think* and how you *feel*—it is not the events that cause you to feel stress and tension, but what you say to yourself about them.

- We are continuously taking in, and evaluating, information about the events occurring around us. These automatic thoughts occur when we react to a situation before we know that we have evaluated it.
- These thoughts, or self-talk, are not planned or intended, they occur quickly, and they may lead to inaccurate perceptions. Self-talk can occur in words, images, and memories, and it can directly influence how we feel.
- If you have ever found yourself in a situation in which you reacted very strongly and you weren't sure why, then you have experienced automatic thoughts. A good example can be seen in the way our parents can "push our buttons"; often, we react without understanding why.
- Monitoring what you say to yourself about internal and external events (your self-talk) can be a powerful tool for changing the way you think.

It is important to understand that it is what you say to yourself about an event that creates your emotions and behavioral reactions to it. Often, people say, "Oh, my husband makes me so mad!" But actually every person creates his or her own feelings by choosing to react a certain way. If you create your feelings, then you also have control over them.

First you need to identify beliefs and attitudes that may cause you to overreact. Many beliefs and attitudes have become so ingrained as a part of ourselves and past experiences that we are no longer even aware of them.

4. Changing Negative Thinking

Thinking errors occur usually without our awareness and can cause us to distort situations and feel unnecessary bad feelings. Try to be open-minded; listen to all of the following thinking errors and see if you have ever experienced any of these either in yourself or in others.

All-or-nothing thinking occurs when you evaluate personal qualifications or situations in extreme, black-or-white categories. For example, before a person developed chronic pain, he may have played baseball. Now he thinks to himself, "If I can't play baseball, I can't enjoy any sport anymore."

- The advantage to thinking this way is that your life seems more predictable, more orderly, and gives you a sense of control.
- The disadvantage of this type of thinking is that our world is full of uncertainty, and living with uncertainty takes time and

experience. The longer that you live accepting life's uncertainties, the more comfortable you are in it.

Overgeneralization happens when you interpret a single negative, such as a romantic rejection or getting fired from your job, as a never-ending pattern of failure that characterizes your life. People who overgeneralize the negative events that occur often feel hopeless and powerless to change the negative events in their lives.

- These can be identified in self-talk that uses words such as *always*, *every time*, or *never*.
- Remember that "misery loves company," and exaggerating your misfortunes will only make you and those around you feel worse.

Mental filtering is a tendency to pick out a single, negative detail and dwell on it exclusively, until you perceive the whole situation as negative. Individuals may focus more intently on negative aspects of an event or give more importance to the negative aspects. An example of this would be the following: You receive positive comments from most of your colleagues after your presentation, but one of them says something mildly critical. Then, you think about their reactions for days and ignore the positive comments.

Discounting the positive is the tendency to take neutral or positive experiences and turn them into negative ones. People can discount positive experiences by minimizing the importance or misinterpreting them as having a negative connotation. If you do a good job, you may insist that anyone could have done it, or that it wasn't good enough. This can make you feel unsatisfied, inadequate, and that your performance is never quite good enough.

Jumping to conclusions happens when we interpret a situation negatively, even though there is no evidence to support this conclusion. Jumping to conclusions can occur in one of two ways: mind reading and fortune telling.

- *Mind reading* is when you assume that you know why someone else does what he or she does, without checking it out first. An example of this is the following: You say "Hi" to a coworker, and he does not respond. You think, "He must be mad at me. I wonder what I did wrong?" When you ask the coworker, he explains that he had been preoccupied with an argument he had earlier with his spouse.
- *Fortune telling* is a tendency to "know" that things are going to turn out badly. Based on your past experiences, you conclude this outcome as an established fact. An example is that you wake up late for work and get stuck in morning traffic. You

say, "Now my whole day is ruined. I'll never get all the things done I need to do today."

Magnification occurs when you exaggerate the importance of a negative event. If you experience a flare-up in pain you may say to yourself, "I can't take this! I can't handle it anymore!" You may not want to handle the pain anymore, and that's okay, but you can stand it.

Minimization is when you do the opposite of magnification: You take personal qualities or events and reduce their importance until they seem insignificant or minimal.

Emotional reasoning is when you assume that reality is the same as your (negative) emotions. You believe that if you feel it, it must be true. An example is when you say to yourself, "I feel worthless." You conclude that you must be a worthless person, or you wouldn't feel that way.

Labeling is an extreme form of all-or-nothing thinking. This refers to identifying a mistake or negative quality and describing an entire situation or individual in terms of that situation. Instead of thinking that you made a mistake, you attach a negative label on yourself, such as "I am a loser/ jerk/failure." For example, a person who suffers from chronic pain might say to herself, "I am defective and without redeeming qualities."

- Labeling a person is irrational; just because you do something that's stupid doesn't mean that you are stupid.
- You must have realistic expectations for yourself. You are only human, and humans make mistakes, and to expect yourself to never make any mistakes just doesn't make sense.

Personalization is when you take on responsibility for a negative event that is beyond your control. An example of this is a mother whose child is having problems in school. Instead of focusing on how to help her child change his problem behaviors, she feels that she must be a bad parent. She obsesses about what her child's behavior means to her and doesn't try to actually solve the problem.

Using *"should" statements* is when you tell yourself that things "should" or "shouldn't" be the way you hoped or expected them to be. They are attempts to motivate by guilt, yourself or others, into behaving in ways that you believe you should.

- "Should" statements directed against yourself can lead to feelings of frustration, guilt, anxiety, or resentment. They also take away your direct control over a situation, as if you are complying with some external authority.
- "Should" statements directed at other people can lead to anger, frustration, or confusion. "Should" statements are negative

thoughts that lead to feelings of frustration about things beyond your control.

5. *The Importance of Communication With One Another*

Everyone has his or her own way of communicating and of determining when and how to express his or her feelings. Communication is a learned set of skills that expresses a message to others and allows you to receive feedback from others.

Communication problems can keep you from expressing your feelings to others. There are three types of communication problems that can block communication.

1. A discrepancy between your words and your wants and needs. This means that there is a difference between what you say you want or need and what you really want. This is remedied by clearly and specifically stating what you want.
2. Failure to express your needs, wants, or feelings to others. Others can't meet your needs if you don't tell them what your needs are.
3. Being a bad listener; this can interrupt communication.

The *attitudes and beliefs* of each person determine when and how they express their feelings. Some attitudes and beliefs may be stopping you from expressing your feelings. Listen with an open mind, and see if you can identify any of these in yourself.

- *Conflict phobia* is when you are afraid of your angry feelings and of facing conflicts with others. You avoid dealing with problems and deny your anger. You may believe that good people don't fight, they are afraid of hurting others, or they think they couldn't handle it if you told them how you really feel.
- *Emotional perfectionism* is a belief that you shouldn't feel irrational feelings, such as anger, jealousy, depression, or anxiety. You believe others would look down on you if they saw weakness or vulnerability in you.
- *Fear of disapproval or of rejection* is when you are afraid others will get mad, or not accept it, if you told them how you really feel. You stuff your feelings down and don't express them, trying to please everyone and meet their expectations of you.
- *Passive–aggressive behavior* is when you fail to express your feelings or needs to others but expect them to know what those needs are. You feel hurt and upset when others don't understand your feelings or meet your needs. Then, you attack them in

subtle, nondirect ways, in an attempt to make them feel guilty. You punish others for not knowing your needs but never tell them why you are upset.

- *Hopelessness* is when you believe a situation won't improve regardless of what you do. You may feel that you have tried everything, or that the other person is unwilling to change. This works as a self-fulfilling prophecy, because if you stop trying to solve the problem, it truly becomes hopeless.
- *Low self-esteem* can interfere with expressing your feelings when you conclude that you aren't entitled to express your feelings or needs to others. You simply go along with others, trying to please them, and meet their expectations, but don't express your needs to others.
- *Spontaneity* is when you give yourself absolute freedom to say anything when you feel upset. Expressing your feelings this way can be hurtful to others and can damage your relationships.
- *Mind reading* is a belief that others will know how you feel or what your needs are, without your ever expressing them. You may feel hurt, neglected, or resentful when others don't meet your needs.
- *Martyrdom* is when you don't express your feelings because you don't want to give anyone the satisfaction of knowing they upset you. You are proud of your ability to hold it in and control your emotions, and you choose to suffer alone in silence.
- *The need to solve problems* can block communication when you focus on finding solutions and don't share your feelings or hear how the other person feels. This leads you to go around the problem without addressing the feelings of those involved.

6. Good Communication Strategies

Good communication strategies include the use of "I" statements, shifting the conversation from talking *about* the other person to talking *to* the other person. Instead of saying, "You make me really angry when you don't call!" say "I feel angry when you don't call!" "I" statements identify your feelings and express them more accurately than "You" statements.

Another good strategy is to discuss the behavior, not the person. Identify the problem behavior specifically; don't accuse the other person as being the problem. It is better to say, "I really feel uptight when you shake your fist at me" than to say, "You really make me feel uptight." Once you have expressed your feelings clearly, listen to the entire message, and then ask questions to clarify any confusions.

7. Relapse Prevention

Following the guidelines and techniques learned during our treatment program, a patient's risk of developing subsequent problems can be reduced by a method called *relapse prevention*. We discuss ways that patients can prepare themselves for stressful times, what to do if they relapse, and signals that identify when they are at risk to relapse into their old behavior. We highlight the following facts for them.

- Remember that these changes should be progressive changes aimed at creating a healthier and happier lifestyle for them and that small mishaps do not equal disaster. Also, if they slip back into unhealthy patterns, they have the power to stop them before they get out of control.
- There are several ways that they can gain control over their unhealthy behaviors. Using the coping strategies that they learned in the program will help them reduce their tension and realistically address their problems.
- Slip-ups are natural for anyone who is attempting to make a lifestyle change, and they should not beat themselves up if they have some problems.
- These slip-ups can be used as a part of their learning process that assists them in making a change in their lifestyle. Identify situations that create, a high risk for, say, craving a cigarette. Situations that evoke stress, are unexpected, or that they know may tempt them to return to their old patterns of behavior should be avoided or approached cautiously.
- Once they have identified these situations, think of ways that they could cope with them in more adaptive and healthy ways.
- Sometimes people try these suggestions learned in the program but are still unable to resolve their problems without some help. In these situations, they can attend a "booster session" that allows them to come to the clinic for a follow-up session to refocus their compliance to this program's guidelines and begin living a healthier lifestyle.
- If they are unable to physically come to the clinic, we can provide them with a telephone interview that will refresh them with the program guidelines and the skills learned.
- Remember that if they find themselves slipping up or returning to old unhealthy patterns, they should not feel embarrassed or give up hope. Contact us, and we will arrange for them to come in and attend a booster session to refresh their memory. Reviewing the sessions in the handbook that we provide them

is another effective way to refresh their memory about the skills learned in these sessions.

8. *Question-and-Answer Period*

Note. From *Psychological Approaches to Pain Management* (2nd ed.), by D. C. Turk and R. J. Gatchel (Eds.), 2002, New York: Guilford Press. Copyright 2002 by Guilford Press. Reprinted with permission.

APPENDIX 3.3

Major Components of the Minimal-Therapist-Contact Treatment

Patient Education

- Provide an orientation overview of the treatment process.
- Explain the rationale for the minimal-therapist-contact treatment approach to headache.
- Emphasize that treatment involves an active role on the part of the patient in collaboration with the therapist.
- Give homework assignments and home-based treatment.
- Develop realistic expectations for treatment outcome.

Therapist Attitude

- Review patient's performance with optimism, magnifying small successes and minimizing any problems as manageable phases of treatment.
- Encourage patients to take credit for their successes, reminding them that they do the difficult work and the therapist primarily acts as a teacher or coach.

Relaxation

- Introduce patient to abdominal breathing exercises.
- Begin progressive muscle relaxation (PMR) training, with practice in tension-release cycles in order to relax the entire body. Patients are requested to practice PMR at least once or twice a day (in the morning and again in the afternoon or the evening). Patients are requested to keep records of their home practice and provide relaxation ratings before and after practice, using a 0–100 point rating scale.
- Consider introducing muscle stretching exercises to strengthen and lengthen sore and tight pericranial muscles.
- Teach muscle scanning and quick relaxation techniques that will enable the patient to rapidly evoke the relaxation response that was learned during PMR training.

- Request that the patient practices abdominal or diaphragmatic breathing for 5–10 min, twice per day. Patients are also asked to subvocalize the word *relax* with each exhalation as they attend to the rhythm of their breathing.
- Teach guided imagery in which a pleasant relaxing image is visualized while the patient is relaxing.
- Teach cue-control relaxation, in which the patient learns to use a cue or signal, such as the word *relax*, when initiating the relaxation practice.
- Use autogenetic training to control the "mental traffic" of patients who may be affected by racing, negative automatic thoughts.

Identifying Early Warning Signs in Headache Patients

- Patients become alerted to common headache triggers and early warning signs or prodromal symptoms that they have recorded in their headache diaries. This provides valuable information to allow patients to take more direct, effective action to prevent or manage their headache.
- Patients are assisted in systematically recording possible prodromal symptoms and in evaluating significance. These symptoms may be psychological, common neurological, or general physiological.
- It is explained to patients that headache precipitants are not universal and do not necessarily also precipitate an attack on every exposure. Headaches may actually occur hours after exposure to a headache trigger.
- Because stress is frequently identified as a headache precipitant, patients are taught to use relaxation techniques and cognitive–behavioral interventions to deal with stress.
- Sleep difficulties, such as insufficient sleep, oversleeping, or irregular sleep schedules, are usually identified as the most common sleep precipitants of headaches. Patients are instructed in proper sleep hygiene and are advised to maintain a regular sleep schedule.
- Hormonal factors, such as reproductive hormones, are often associated with headache disorders, particularly migraine. Making patients more aware of their increased susceptibility during periods such as menstruation is important.
- Meal schedules and dietary factors are often closely associated with headaches, especially migraine headaches. Dietary factors, such as skipping or delaying meals or ingesting specific foods,

beverages, or ingredients, can often trigger headaches. Migraine patients should be advised to consume alcohol, particularly red wine, with caution and eliminate monosodium glutamate, aspartame, and nitrites from their diets. The role of caffeine as a potential precipitant of headaches should also be explored.

- Environmental factors (e.g., air pollution, weather changes, barometric pressure changes, perfumes/colognes, noise, motion, exposure to vapors or chemicals) should also be discussed with patients, because such factors can be headache triggers.

Effective Use of Headache Medications

- A careful assessment of appropriate medications that can be effective in dealing with symptoms, as well as preventive medications, should be carefully explored with the patients.
- A discussion of "rebound headaches" in response to medication should be provided.

Responding to Early Warning Signs and Triggers

- The information collected from the headache diaries will provide a list of headache warning signs and triggers.
- A RESCUE plan is developed for each patient in response to these early warning signs and triggers: Remain calm, Escape from known triggers, Stay away from stress or stressful situations, Carry your medications with you at all times, Use relaxation exercises, Eat and sleep on schedule.

Cognitive–Behavioral Stress-Management

- Stress management is an important headache management skill, because stress is the most frequently reported headache trigger.
- Cognitive–behavioral therapy is beneficial for dealing with psychosocial stressors, maladaptive thoughts and behaviors, and stress-generating beliefs.

Thermal Biofeedback

- The goal is to teach patients to warm their hands through volitional peripheral vasodilation, with the assistance of thermal biofeedback.
- It is important for patients to develop this sense of internal control because it will enhance their perception of control over the headaches.

Pain Management

The same relaxation and stress management skills used to prevent headaches can also be used during headache episodes in order to manage the pain.

Maintenance of Self-Management

- Emphasize to patients that once they develop control over their headaches, maintenance of these gains will require continued effort.
- Plan posttreatment strategies to maintain therapeutic gains.
- Remind patients that an occasional "checkup" or booster sessions may be needed in the event of some momentary relapse.

Note. From "Cognitive–Behavior Management of Recurrent Headache Disorders: A Minimal-Therapist-Contact Approach," by G. L. Lipchik, K. A. Holroyd, and J. M. Nash, in *Psychological Approaches to Pain Management: A Practitioner's Handbook* (2nd ed., pp. 365–389), edited by D. C. Turk and R. J. Gatchel, 2002, New York: Guilford Press. Copyright 2002 by Guilford Press. Adapted with permission.

APPENDIX 3.4A

Steps in Learning to Relax: An Overview

During subsequent sessions of treatment, you will be taught some relaxation exercises, and may be given an audiocassette so that you can practice at home.

- *Eliminate distractions.* Initially, the place where you practice should be quiet, comfortable, and free of distractions. Unplug the telephone, turn off the television, close the door, and so on.
- *Find a comfortable chair.* A recliner is best because your entire body is supported and muscular tension is reduced. If you do not have a recliner, you may use a high-backed chair with a stool or a sofa.
- *Get comfortable.* Remove constricting clothing, shoes, and glasses or contact lenses, and loosen your belt.
- *Go with the process.* Learning to relax is somewhat different than learning most other activities. Rather than "trying harder," you must adopt the idea of going with the process. Just let it happen. Unusual feelings like tingling in the fingers or floating sensations are signs that the muscles are beginning to loosen. Do not worry if you actually feel more tense after the first practice session.
- *Remember that success may vary from day to day.* The ability to relax will vary from day to day, depending on the state of your

body and mind due to lack of sleep, diet, premenstrual tension, work overload, illness, and so on, so do not worry if initially the relaxation exercises don't always help reduce anxiety.

- *Make practice part of your daily routine.* If you are too busy to practice on most days, then you are too busy.
- *Find your best time to practice.* After work and before bedtime seem to be the most popular times to practice, but pick times when you are neither too rushed nor too tired.

Relaxation Exercises

1. What is a relaxation exercise?
   - When you go somewhere by yourself, get in a comfortable position, close your eyes, and allow yourself to get deeply relaxed for 20 min, 30 min, or more (depending on how long it takes you).
   - This does not mean that you go to sleep.
   - Some different ways of doing a relaxation exercise are the following:
     - listening to a relaxation tape;
     - body scanning (scanning down through all the different parts of your body);
     - just focusing on maintaining a smooth, even breathing pattern;
     - meditating (repeating a word or phrase over and over); and
     - imagery (creating pleasant and relaxing scenes in your mind).
2. What are you trying to accomplish when you practice a relaxation exercise?
   - Relax your body and mind.
   - Increase your body awareness (your ability to identify and release tension in your body).
   - Train your focus (your ability to move your mind away from worries and pain).
3. When should you do a relaxation exercise?
   - When you're stressed or tense.
   - When you're having trouble going to sleep.
   - When your pain flares up.
4. How can relaxation exercises help pain?
   - By reducing muscle tension and stress in your body that can cause or increase pain.
   - By calming down emotions that can increase your pain.
   - By focusing your mind away from pain.

- Remember, when your pain is very intense, it will take longer to have success with your relaxation exercise, so you need to remind yourself to be patient (it may take 45 min, or an hour, or more, until your pain calms down).
5. How often should you practice relaxation exercises (with the tape or just on your own)?
   - Practice with the tape until you can feel that you can have some success without the tape.
   - Practice your breathing technique (eyes closed, no distractions, for 5 or 10 min or longer) until you can maintain a smooth, even breathing pattern without your mind wandering off too much.
   - Eventually, you may be doing several things at once during your relaxation exercises, including your breathing, scanning down through your body, repeating relaxing phrases, bringing pleasant images into your mind, and so on.
   - Although relaxation exercises can help you go to sleep, you should find another time during the day to practice them (you can't learn anything when you're asleep).

Note. From *Biofeedback: Methods and Procedures in Clinical Practice,* by G. F. von Bozzay, 1984, San Francisco: Biofeedback Institute of San Francisco. Copyright 1984 by G. F. von Bozzay. Reprinted with permission.

APPENDIX 3.4B

Deep, Diaphragmatic Breathing

Breathing is essential for life. The purpose of breathing is to get oxygen into the body and to get carbon dioxide, a waste product, out of the body. Although we all breathe, few of us retain the habit of natural, full breathing experienced by an infant.

When you take a breath or inhale, air is drawn in through the nose and warmed by the mucous membrane of your nasal passages. The bristly hairs of your nostrils filter out impurities, which are expelled when you breathe out, or exhale. The lungs have no muscles of their own for breathing and rely on the diaphragm, the dome-shaped muscle that separates the chest cavity from the abdominal cavity, to expand and contract for breathing. During inhalation, the diaphragm flattens downward to create more space in the chest cavity, allowing the lungs to fill more completely. During exhalation, the diaphragm relaxes and returns to its dome shape.

Diaphragmatic breathing is based on methods that have been practiced for thousands of years for achieving calmness and reduction of tension. It involves learning to use the diaphragm, rather than the shoulder and chest muscles, to draw air into the lungs. This allows more efficient breathing with less muscular work. It allows you to relax the neck and shoulder muscles while breathing.

Training Procedures for Diaphragmatic Breathing

- *A recliner.* A recliner or high-backed chair with arms is ideal, because the entire body is supported and muscular tension is reduced.
- *Hand placement.* Place your right hand on your stomach, between the bottom of your rib cage and your navel. Place your left hand on your chest, on your breastbone, just below your collarbone.
- *Baseline breathing.* Now just breathe regularly, through your nose, and notice the rise and fall of your hands as you inhale and exhale.
- *Diaphragmatic practice.* As you inhale, imagine your stomach to be a balloon that inflates, lifting your right hand. As you exhale, the balloon deflates, and your right hand falls. Your left hand remains still as your right hand rises and falls.
- *Feedback.* Do not try to force it; just attend to the motion of your hands and the feelings in your chest. Allow your right hand to rise and fall while your left hand remains still. (Some people find it helpful to imagine their right hand is a boat, rising and falling on the slow, rolling waves of the ocean, while their left hand sits quietly on the dock.)
- *Slow breathing.* Next, slow your breathing by pausing very briefly at the top and bottom of each breath. Pause for just a second or so—do not hold your breath or pause so long that you are uncomfortable.
- *Tension release.* Notice how there is a slight increase in tension as you breathe in, and a decrease as you breathe out. Concentrate on the tension flowing out with each breath. Feel a slight increase in tension as you inhale, and then let go as you exhale. Each time you exhale, feel the tension leaving your body. Let your whole body become limp all over and allow it to sink deep in your chair.
- *Placement of hands at sides.* After one or two sessions with your hands on your chest and abdomen, your hands can usually be placed on the arms of the chair or in your lap.
- *Some difficulties.* For most people, diaphragmatic breathing is awkward and uncomfortable at first. Like learning any new skill, with consistent practice most people can become proficient and comfortable with this new style of breathing.

Some Additional Things to Always Keep in Mind When You Practice

- *Breathe slowly*. When you are using your breathing for relaxation and pain control, you will want to breathe slowly and more deeply than you normally breathe. If you find that it is hard to slow down, then try pursing your lips when you exhale, like you're blowing out a candle, and focus on breathing out slowly on each breath.
- *Breathe into your stomach*. Breath into your stomach so that your stomach fills up like a balloon. When you breathe out, just allow the air to escape slowly from your stomach like you're letting air out of the balloon.
- *Don't strain*. Let your breathing feel comfortable. Don't force your breathing. If it feels like you're straining, then back off. Deep breathing should help calm you down; it should not require a lot of effort or increase tension.
- *Keep it moving*. One of the main goals is to keep a smooth, even breathing pattern going. At first, you may have difficulty staying focused, keeping your mind on your breathing, or keeping it in rhythm. Every time your mind wanders, just notice that it has wandered and gently bring it back to your breathing pattern.
- *Maintain a rhythm*. If you have difficulty maintaining a steady rhythm, try repeating something in your mind along with your breathing. For instance, try counting to 4 on each inhale and 4 on each exhale; or try saying the words "breathing in" and "breathing out" in your mind. You can also try using a mental image that has rhythm, such as watching ocean waves roll up onto the beach and roll back into the surf.

Suggestions for Relaxing With Your Breathing

- Think about breathing in feelings of relaxation and breathing out feelings of tension.
- Let your whole body relax a little bit more each time you breathe out.
- Allow your body to feel like it's sinking down.
- Allow your shoulders to droop down.
- Let your jaw feel loose.
- Imagine that your arms and legs feel heavy and comfortable.
- Let the muscles in your face smooth out.
- Remind yourself to calm down several times.

Note. From *Biofeedback: Methods and Procedures in Clinical Practice*, by G. F. von Bozzay, 1984, San Francisco: Biofeedback Institute of San Francisco. Copyright 1984 by G. F. von Bozzay. Reprinted with permission.

APPENDIX 3.4C

Abbreviated Progressive Muscle Relaxation Training

The following are general guidelines for an abbreviated muscle relaxation training procedure:

1. Instruct the patient to "make a fist with your dominant hand [usually right]. Make a fist and tense the muscles of your [right] hand and forearm; tense until it trembles. Feel the muscles pull across your fingers and the lower part of your forearm." Have the patient hold this position for 5 to 7 seconds; then say "relax," instructing him or her to just let his or her hand go: "Pay attention to the muscles of your [right] hand and forearm as they relax. Note how those muscles feel as relaxation flows through them" (10–20 seconds).

   "Again, tense the muscles of your [right] hand and forearm. Pay attention to the muscles involved" (5–7 seconds). "OK, relax; attend only to those muscles, and note how they feel as the relaxation takes place, becoming more and more relaxed, more relaxed than ever before. Each time we do this you'll relax even more until your arm and hand are completely relaxed with no tension at all, warm and relaxed."

   Continue until the patient reports that his or her (right) hand and forearm are completely relaxed, with no tension (usually two to four times is sufficient).

2. Instruct the patient to tense his or her (right) biceps, leaving his or her hand and forearm on the chair. Proceed in the same manner as above, in a hypnotic monotone, using the (right) hand as a reference point (i.e., move on when the patient reports that his or her biceps feel as completely relaxed as his or her hand and forearm).

   Proceed to other gross-muscle groups (listed below) in the same manner, with the same verbalization; for example: "Note how these muscles feel as they relax; feel the relaxation and warmth flow through these muscles; pay attention to these muscles so that later you can relax them again." Always use the preceding group as a reference for moving on.

   - Nondominant (left) hand and forearm—feel muscles over knuckles and on lower part of arm.
   - Nondominant (left) biceps.
   - Frown hard, tensing muscles of forehead and top of head (these muscles often "tingle" as they relax).

- Wrinkle nose, feeling muscles across top of cheeks and upper lip.
- Draw corners of mouth back, feeling jaw muscles and cheeks.
- Tighten chin and throat muscles, feeling two muscles in front of throat.
- Tighten chest muscles and muscles across back—feel muscles pull below shoulder blades.
- Tighten abdominal muscles—make abdomen hard.
- Tighten muscles of right upper leg—feel one muscle on top and two on the bottom of the upper leg.
- Tighten right calf—feel muscles on bottom of right calf.
- Push down with toes and arch right foot—feel pressure as if something were pushing up under the arch.
- Tighten left upper leg.
- Tighten left calf.
- Tighten left foot.

For most muscle groups, two presentations will suffice. Ask the patient if he or she feels any tension anywhere in his or her body. If he or she does, go back and repeat the tension-release cycle for that muscle group. It is often helpful to instruct the patient to take a deep breath and hold it while tensing muscles and to let it go while releasing. Should any muscle group not respond after four trials, move on and return to it later.

Keep in mind the following caution: Some patients may develop muscle cramps or spasms from prolonged tension of muscles. If this occurs, shorten the tension interval a few seconds, and instruct the patient not to tense muscles quite so hard.

Although the word *hypnosis* is not to be used, progressive relaxation, properly executed, does seem to create a state resembling a light hypnotic trance state, with the individual more susceptible to suggestion. Relaxation may be further deepened by repetition of suggestions of warmth, relaxation, and so on. Some patients may actually report sensations of disassociation from their bodies. This is complete relaxation and is to be expected. Patients should be instructed to speak as little as possible while under relaxation.

In bringing participants back to "normal," use the numerical method of trance termination: "I'm going to count from 1 to 4. On the count of 1, start moving your legs; 2, your fingers and hands; 3, your head; and 4, open your eyes and sit up. One—move your legs; two—now your fingers and hands; three—move your head around; four—open your eyes and sit up." Always check to see that the patient feels well, alert, and so on, before leaving.

The patient should be instructed to practice relaxation twice a day between sessions. He or she should not work at it more than 15 min at a time and should not practice twice within any 3-hr period. He or she should practice alone. Relaxation may be used for getting to sleep if practiced while the patient is horizontal; if he or she does not wish to sleep, then he or she should practice sitting up. Relaxation, properly timed, can be used to rejuvenate one for the rest of the day.

By the third session, if the patient has been practicing well, relaxation may be induced merely by focusing attention on the muscle groups and instructing the patient to "concentrate on muscles becoming relaxed, warm," and so on. However, if the patient has difficulty following straight suggestions, return to the use of tension-release techniques.

Note. From *Biofeedback: Methods and Procedures in Clinical Practice,* by G. F. von Bozzay, 1984, San Francisco: Biofeedback Institute of San Francisco. Copyright 1984 by G. F. von Bozzay. Reprinted with permission.

APPENDIX 3.4D

Passive Relaxation: An Overview

Stress and tension can interfere with your ability to control pain and can keep you from enjoying things that you normally would. Stress and tension can cause fatigue and increased pain. They are normal reactions that have evolved from our natural fight-or-flight response, which occurs when a situation is perceived as threatening. A certain level of tension is needed to function effectively, but often our tension level exceeds this. Scientific and clinical studies have demonstrated that relaxation is effective in the management of pain.

Today we will learn relaxation techniques and how you can apply them to help manage your pain. When beginning relaxation, it is important to recognize your body's signals of tension and become aware of your tension sites. Relaxation can be used to combat the effects of tension and stress on our bodies and when we are confronted with a stress-producing situation. Identify situations that are particularly stressful for you. Once identified, schedule relaxation practice before entering the situation to help you remain calm and relaxed. If you are unsure of when they occur, ask yourself "Are there any specific times of the day in which I tend to feel more tense?" The Daily Pain Log (see Exhibit 3.1B) can be effective in assessing the times of the day and the situations that surround your pain. This information can be found in the Remarks section of the Daily Pain Log to identify any situational pattern in regard to pain. Relaxing before potentially stressful situations, and during more tense times of the day, will help reduce your overall tension. Consistent relaxation practice will help identify when you are becoming tense and will help you to relax.

In unexpected stressful situations, mini-relaxation sessions should be used, in which you pay attention to your body's tension level and intervene at the earliest point. To determine your tension level, focus on the muscle group that usually holds your tension and see if it feels relaxed or tense. When in a stressful situation, take a deep breath and exhale slowly while repeating your own relaxation word. Your relaxation word can be anything you want, but it should be calming and help you relax. Imagery used during relaxation, such as imagining yourself in the situation acting in a calm manner, can be helpful. Don't feel frustrated if relaxation is hard at first, or if you have problems relaxing completely. Remember that you are changing the way you respond to a situation, and it takes time, practice, and patience.

During relaxation training, expect slow but gradual progress, and give yourself credit for all progress achieved. Relaxation, like any other skill, must be practiced, and it will improve if you practice consistently. Don't expect an immediate change; it will take time to change behaviors that you have had for so long, and remember that everybody will differ in how quickly they learn to relax.

Passive Relaxation Procedure

I want you to find a comfortable chair and make whatever minor adjustments you need to make to *allow* yourself to be as comfortable and unrestricted as possible. Now, allow your mind to just *drift* throughout your body and check that everything is loose and relaxed and that no part of your body feels restricted or uncomfortable. Make whatever *minor adjustments* you need to make now to allow yourself to be in a most comfortable position.

Now, just begin your deep, diaphragmatic breathing. Notice the rise and fall as you inhale and exhale. As you inhale, imagine your stomach to be a boat that floats, rising and falling. As you inhale, the boat rises on the wave. Do not try to force it. Just attend to the motion and the feelings in your chest. Now, slow your breathing by pausing very briefly at the top and bottom of each breath. Just pause a second or so. Do not hold your breath or pause so you are uncomfortable. Notice how there is a slight increase in tension as you breathe in and a decrease as you breathe out. Concentrate on the tension as you inhale, and then let go as you exhale. Each time you exhale, feel the tension leaving your body. Let your whole body become limp all over and allow it to sink deep in your chair. Now, allow your attention to just drift to the very top of your head, to your forehead and scalp. Smooth out all the muscles in your forehead and scalp. Just let them go, relax them. *Smooth* those muscles out and let your scalp rest very comfortably on top of your head. Allow this relaxation to just *flow* down over your eyebrows, eyelids, even relaxing the back of your eyes, letting your eyes rest quite comfortably. *Continue* to let the relaxation flow over your whole face—your cheeks, lips, and chin, letting your whole face become very comfortably heavy and relaxed. Now, *pay special attention* to your jaw, allowing the muscles that hold up your jaw to relax—just let them go. You might notice that your jaw will be pulled down slightly by gravity. As that happens, your lips will part slightly. As you continue to relax your face and jaw, also let go of your tongue, throat, and your vocal chords. Allow your vocal chords to become quite quiet and relaxed, with your tongue resting very comfortably on the floor of your mouth.

Let this relaxation continue to flow down the back of your head, and let go of all the muscles around your neck and down your shoulders. *Smooth* out all the muscles of your neck and shoulders. You might even think of them as tiny knotted rope that you untie and let hang loose and limp. Smooth them out and just let them hang loose, limp and relaxed. Now, also continue to relax your shoulders and neck muscles and allow that relaxation to flow down into your arms, relaxing all the muscles of your upper arm down to your elbows and your forearms. Smooth out all those muscles and let them go. Let go of the muscles around your wrists and hands, all the way down to your fingertips, letting your arms become comfortably heavy and relaxed. As your arms become more and more relaxed and heavy, let the blood flow more comfortably into your fingertips and realize, as you let go of the tension in your arms and shoulders, that the blood flows more comfortably and easily into the fingertips.

As you continue to relax your head and face, your neck and shoulders and your arms, let your attention now drift to the upper back, and smooth out all the muscles along your shoulders and upper back. Continue to relax all the way along your spine, down your middle back, smoothing out all the muscles and down into your lower back, letting go all the way down into your waist. Allow this relaxation to come around the sides of your body, letting go of all the muscles around your ribcage, smoothing them out and letting go. With every breath, allow your chest to become more and more comfortably relaxed. Just observe your breathing with every breath. Notice the inhalation of the air through your nostrils, down, down into your lungs, filling up the lungs and then exhaling back out again and allow your breathing to be just normal, rhythmic, smooth. With every breath, allow yourself just to float down into that chair. Let the relaxation spread down to your abdomen, your waist, smoothing out all the muscles in your stomach to become quite relaxed. Just notice and feel this relaxed, peaceful breathing.

Now, also relax all the muscles around your hips, waist, and pelvis, letting your whole pelvic area relax and smooth out. Continue to let that relaxation flow down to your thighs, knees, down to your shins, calves, letting your legs become quite heavy, comfortably heavy and relaxed. Let go of your ankles, heels, feet—even the soles of your feet and toes. As your legs become comfortably heavy, blood flows again more easily to the toes, allowing your feet to become comfortably warm.

Your whole body, from the very top of your head all the way down to the ends of your toes, is now relaxed, peacefully calm, quite quiet inside. With every breath now, allow your body to let go a little bit more. With every exhalation, let your body just float on down through the chair, comfortably heavy and relaxed. As you relax more and more and more deeply, remain *awake and aware*, but very relaxed. Relaxation allows the whole system to have a very deep rest while you are awake and aware. Relaxation is *different from tiredness*. Whereas tiredness is a drain of energy produced by too much tension in the system, relaxation allows you to *conserve the energy* that was formerly used up by tension through deep relaxation, such as you are experiencing now. The body can get a very deep rest and you can feel *refreshed* and *rejuvenated*.

As you practice these techniques of deep progressive relaxation realize that, as with any other *skill*, you become more and *more capable* and effective at *relaxing more quickly* and more *efficiently*, so that soon, rather than going through the entire process, muscle group by muscle group, the words *calm*, *quite quiet*, or *relaxed* will allow you to achieve the same quality of deep relaxation that you are experiencing now and, with practice, the depth of relaxation can also be increased.

Note. From *Biofeedback: Methods and Procedures in Clinical Practice*, by G. F. von Bozzay, 1984, San Francisco: Biofeedback Institute of San Francisco. Copyright 1984 by G. F. von Bozzay. Reprinted with permission.

APPENDIX 3.5

Biofeedback Therapy

What is Biofeedback?

- It is a learning technique.
- Processes that are happening in your body are measured and displayed to you by biofeedback equipment.
- Some of the things that are measured with the biofeedback equipment are muscle tension, breathing pattern, and hand temperature. (Did you know that your hands tend to get warmer when you are more relaxed, and cooler when you are more stressed?)

What Will I Be Doing in My Biofeedback Therapy Sessions?

- Biofeedback training with the biofeedback equipment.
- Taking stress management classes.

- Learning and practicing relaxation exercises (which are used to control stress and pain).

How Can Biofeedback Therapy Help Me?

- You can learn to be more aware of areas of tension in your body. Most people have areas of tension in their body of which they are not aware.
- You can learn to relax better and release tension from your body.
- You can learn to have more control over the stress in your life.
- You can learn some ways of getting your pain to calm down when it flares up.
- You can learn some ways of preventing your pain from flaring up in the first place.

What Is Self-Regulation?

Think of your body as a car and your nervous system as a car engine; you are the driver. When driving a car, you need a burst of energy to get onto the highway, and you let your engine idle while sitting at a stoplight, and you turn it off when you get home. You make similar demands on your body. A good deal of stress may be needed to successfully meet a critical deadline at work, less stress is needed to carry on a conversation with a group of friends, and very little stress is required to sit quietly and read a book. Just like your body, the harder, faster, and longer you drive your car, the quicker different parts will wear out or break. By using only the amount of gas you need, you can conserve energy and increase the life of your car and your body. By learning some simple relaxation techniques, and using them all through the day, you can learn to *self-regulate* the amount of stress and tension in your body and keep your pain from flaring up. It is important to remember that if you have been suffering with pain for a long time, you may not be aware of all the stress and tension in your body.

There are many ways to self-regulate stress and tension during the day. Breathing, body scanning, and monitoring bad habits are three techniques that you will learn in biofeedback therapy.

II
ASSESSING AND TREATING PAIN

4

THE STEPWISE APPROACH TO
PAIN EVALUATION

> The investigator who would study pain is at the mercy of the patient,
> upon whose ability and willingness to communicate he is dependent.
> —L. Lasagna (1960)

Before any attempt is made at pain management intervention, assessment is essential. As I have reviewed elsewhere (Gatchel, 2000), most health care professionals are under time constraints, as well as billing constraints imposed by third-party payers, when deciding the best method of evaluating patients with pain. Therefore, a frequently asked question is the following: "If I were to choose the most time- and cost-efficient assessment method, which one should I select?" Unfortunately, one needs to avoid the assumption that there is a single instrument that can serve as the best assessment. For many patients, several assessments will be needed. Rather than asking which instrument should be used, a better question is: "What sequence of testing should I consider to develop the best understanding of potential biopsychosocial problems that might be encountered with this patient?"

Assessment should proceed from a global biopsychosocial diagnosis of pain to a more detailed evaluation of the most important interactive factors of this diagnosis. There are numerous biological measurement and diagnosis methods that can be used (Woessner, 2003). Of course, it is initially important to provide patients with a brief overview of the concept of pain. Providing a brochure to patients is often helpful in reinforcing what is said face to face. Appendix 4.2 presents a brief brochure my colleagues and I often use when treating back pain patients in our interdisciplinary pain management program. This can serve as a prototype for developing similar ones for other pain disorders.

As Gatchel and Oordt (2003) pointed out, it is important to distinguish pain as a neurological event from pain perception. The neurological event is called *nociception*, which originates in pain receptors/regions and then passes through nerve fibers and pathways to the central nervous system. *Pain perception* is the actual interpretation of pain sensation by the patient. This often can be a two-way pathway; that is, the perception of the nociceptive event can significantly influence one's emotional and behavioral response. The stress associated with the meaning of pain, in turn, can then have a significant effect on the original nociception by decreasing pain threshold. Indeed, oftentimes various pain syndromes can lead to pressures and changes of lifestyle that most people find unpleasant, at the very least. Unplanned and unwanted lifestyle changes can lead to stress, so patients may begin to feel worse than they anticipated, and the stress actually can interfere with physical recovery. This can be explained in terms of a cycle in which pain and the changes that it brings lead to stress, which leads to increased pain, which leads to increased stress, and so on. I reviewed this *pain–stress cycle* and its effect on the hypothalamic–pituitary–adrenal axis in chapter 1. Indeed, many studies have demonstrated that stress and anxiety significantly influence pain perception, with higher levels of stress or anxiety associated with higher levels of pain intensity (Cornwal & Doncieri, 1988). Moreover, stress may activate biological responses in the autonomic and musculoskeletal systems. Thus, for example, muscle spasms may occur with the anxiety accompanying tension headaches which, in turn, produces more pain and muscle tension, and so on. This *pain–stress cycle*, presented in chapter 2, Figure 2.1, can often be important to point out to patients. Also, as I reviewed in chapter 1, the gate-control model of pain should be presented to patients in order to provide them with a better conceptualization of the pain mechanism process.

THE STEPWISE APPROACH

Psychosocial and personality assessment should be viewed as a *stepwise approach*, proceeding from global indexes of emotional distress and disturbance to more detailed evaluations of specific diagnoses of Axis I Clinical and Axis II Personality Disorders. Figure 4.1 is a flowchart for such a process. It should be noted that specific assessment tools have been developed for many types of pain disorders, including the Roland and Morris Disability Questionnaire for Chronic Low Back Pain (Roland & Morris, 1983) and the Research Diagnostic Criteria for Temporomandibular Disorders (Dworkin &

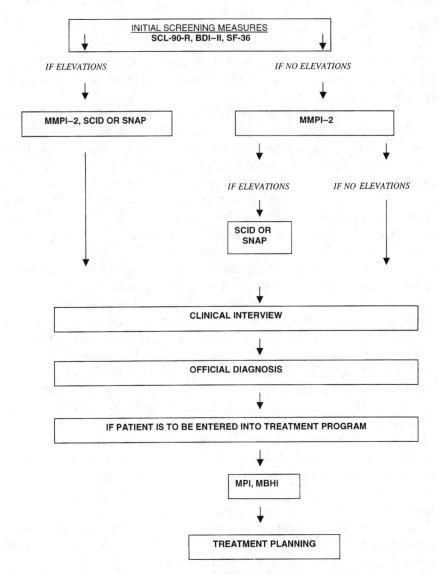

Figure 4.1. Diagnostic process for delineating psychosocial and personality characteristics of pain patients. For some disorders, there also could be a specific assessment tool developed that would be administered at this time. SCL-90-R = Symptom Checklist–90–Revised; BDI–II = Beck Depression Inventory—II; SF-36 = Short Form–36; MMPI–2 = Minnesota Multiphasic Personality Inventory—2; SCID: Structured Clinical Interview for *DSM* Diagnoses; SNAP = Schedule for Nonadaptive and Adaptive Personality; MPI = Multidimensional Pain Inventory; MBHI = Millon Behavioral Health Inventory. From "How Practitioners Should Evaluate Personality to Help Manage Patients With Chronic Pain," by R. J. Gatchel, in *Personality Characteristics of Patients With Pain*, edited by R. J. Gatchel and J. N. Weisberg, 2000, Washington, DC: American Psychological Association. Copyright 2000 by the American Psychological Association. Reprinted with permission.

LeResche, 1992). Turk and Melzack (1992, 2001) and I (Gatchel, 2001) have provided detailed source books of various specific assessment instruments. These evaluation tools, which address particular issues associated with specific pain conditions, should be used in addition to the diagnostic process delineated in Figure 4.1.

An initial screening process to flag obvious psychological distress, which can be done efficiently via the mail, even before seeing the patient, might be sending out a brief questionnaire (soliciting information about major stressors or life changes that are occurring, degree of emotional distress, work status, etc.) and having the patient send it back before the first visit. The first session then might consist of the administration of the Beck Depression Inventory—II (BDI–II; Beck, Brown, & Steer, 1996), the Symptom Check List–90–Revised (SCL-90-R; Derogatis, 1994) and the Short Form–36 (SF-36; Ware, Snow, Kosinski, & Gandek, 1993). Pronounced scale elevations on these instruments would alert clinical staff to the degree of emotional distress or dysfunction in a pain patient and indicate the need for a more thorough evaluation. This would subsequently include the administration of the Minnesota Multiphasic Personality Inventory—2 (MMPI–2; Butcher, Dahlstrom, Graham, Tellegen, & Kaemmer, 1989) as well as the Structured Clinical Interview for DSM Diagnosis (SCID; First, Spitzer, Gibbon, & Williams, 1995) or the Schedule of Nonadaptive and Adaptive Personality (SNAP; Clark, 1993). The SCID can be administered only if trained personnel are available; the SNAP is a self-report instrument. If no pronounced elevations were displayed on the BDI–II, SCL-90-R, and SF-36, the MMPI–2 would still be administered, because third-party payers are accustomed to having this widely accepted test as part of a pain evaluation. If there were no meaningful profile elevations on the MMPI–2, then one could proceed directly to a clinical interview. If elevations on the MMPI–2 were exhibited, then the SCID or the SNAP would be administered. Administration of either one supports an official *Diagnostic and Statistical Manual of Mental Disorders* (American Psychiatric Association, 1994) based diagnosis of an Axis I or Axis II disorder.

The Clinical Interview

The next step is administration of a psychosocial clinical interview, which is a powerful assessment tool of the clinician. A brief screening checklist, as well as a mini mental status examination, is quite helpful (see Appendix 4.3). The mini mental status examination will immediately alert the clinician to patient disorientation and possible cognitive impairment. Obviously, such impairment may invalidate basic testing in general, perhaps prompting referral for a neuropsychological evaluation. In addition to the traditional areas explored in a clinical history, there are other areas that should be explored with patients, especially if the pain is chronic. The structured psychosocial–personality test results will sensitize the clinician to what needs attention. Some issues that are important to cover in a clinical interview consist of the following potential barriers to recovery that could affect response to treatment:

- patient and family history of mental health, such as depression and substance abuse;
- history of head injury, convulsions, or impairment of function;
- any stressful changes in lifestyle or marital status before or since the injury that precipitated the pain;
- work history, including explanation of job losses, changes, and dissatisfaction;
- financial history, contrasting current income with past, and comparing these with current cost-of-living requirements; and
- any litigation or workers' compensation claim pending for the patient's current medical and pain problem.

In addition to the above, the determination of the patient's motivation for change is another important, if unstated, purpose of the interview process. Many chronic-pain patients restrict their lives by avoiding any risk of experiencing pain, through immobilization and use of analgesics. Patients who actively engage in pain management program requirements clearly have suspect motivation for change. Jensen (1996) provided an excellent review of methods for enhancing patient motivation in pain treatment programs, which I present in chapter 7. Finally, it should also be pointed out that this initial assessment provides the opportunity to start educating patients about pain mechanisms.

The clinical interview allows the clinician to contrast the patient's current psychosocial functioning with past functioning and to compare the testing data with the interview data. The clinician can then estimate the potential for getting the patient to change behavior and work toward rehabilitation. Finally, with this clinical assessment material in hand, if it is decided that the patient is a suitable candidate to enter a comprehensive pain management program, an additional set of assessment instruments should be administered: the Multidimensional Pain Inventory (MPI; Kerns, Turk, & Rudy, 1985) and the Millon Behavioral Health Inventory (MBHI; Millon, Green, & Meagher, 1982). These instruments are beneficial for treatment personnel, who can use the results to identify the best approach for pain management and to anticipate potential problems in the pain management program. It should also be noted that Millon and colleagues have recently developed the Millon Behavioral Medicine Diagnostic (Millon, Antoni, Millon, & Davis, 2003) which has some newer advantages over the MBHI.

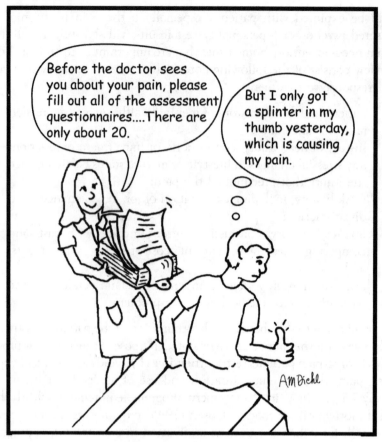

The way not to take a stepwise approach to the assessment of pain.

The Multidimensional Pain Inventory

The MPI, also known as the *West Haven–Yale Multidimensional Pain Inventory* (Kerns et al., 1985), was initially developed to measure three psychological dimensions of pain: (a) patient self-reported pain and the effect of that pain, (b) response of significant others to the communication of pain patients, and (c) level of activities of daily living. The instrument was shown to have good psychometric properties. Turk and Rudy (1988) subsequently developed a classification system based on the MPI, which categorized patients according to three subgroups that predicted response to treatment: (a) *dysfunctional*, (b) *interpersonally distressed*, and (c) *adaptive copers*. According to this classification system, dysfunctional profile patients are hypothesized to *not* respond as well to intervention as would patients in the other two subgroups. Indeed, a study conducted by Asmundson,

Norton, and Alterdings (1997) demonstrated that patients with chronic low back pain who were classified as dysfunctional on the MPI reported more pain-specific fear and avoidance than did patients in the other two subgroups. Such characteristics were, in turn, related to poorer coping ability in these dysfunctional chronic-pain patients.

Turk and Okifuji (1998) reviewed other research demonstrating the utility of the MPI with other chronic-pain conditions, including headache, temporomandibular jaw pain, and fibromyalgia. Assessment of such MPI profiles will help to tailor the needs for treatment strategies to account for the different personality characteristics of patients. For example, patients with an interpersonally distressed profile may need additional clinical attention addressing interpersonal skills to perform effectively in a group-oriented treatment program. Pain patients with dysfunctional and interpersonally distressed profiles display more indications of acute and chronic personality differences relative to adaptive-coper profile patients, and they would therefore require more clinical management (e.g., Etscheidt, Steiger, & Braverman, 1995). Such additional attention, however, would not necessarily be essential for adaptive-coper profile patients.

Studies such as those above support the notion that, because patients' responses to treatment differ as a function of their psychosocial coping profiles, then some specific treatment modalities are more likely to be better suited than others for each profile. An important issue for future clinical research is whether there are other types of biopsychosocial profiles that are more or less responsive to different treatment modalities. For example, variables that have been found to be predictors of pain-related disability outcomes, such as catastrophizing, fear of movement/reinjury, pain beliefs, anxiety, and depression, and their interactions with environmental factors, such as workplace variables, and health care system variables, need to be more closely evaluated.

The Millon Behavioral Health Inventory

Millon et al. (1982) originally developed the MBHI, which is a 150-question true–false test based on 20 clinical scales that reflect medically related concerns, such as compliance with treatment regimens and reaction to treatment personnel. The MBHI's clinical scales include those that rate introversive style, cooperative style, social style, premorbid pessimism, pain treatment responsivity, and emotional vulnerability. Several of these scales are clinically meaningful in the assessment of pain patients. For example, in our treatment programs for patients with chronic low back pain, my colleagues and I often find that people who score low on the Cooperative Style scale and high on the Sensitive Style scale demonstrate poor treatment outcome (Gatchel, Mayer, Capra, Diamond, & Barnett, 1986). These patients usually tend not to follow advice and can be unpredictable and moody. Obviously, such personality characteristics can be detrimental to any group-oriented treatment process. In marked contrast, patients who score high on cooperative and sociable scales demonstrate excellent outcome. My colleagues and I have also found that patients who score high on the Emotional Vulnerability scale usually require additional psychological treatment in dealing with their pain and disability, as we have found in treating chronic-headache patients (Gatchel, Deckel, Weinberg, & Smith, 1985). The MBHI scales can be useful for helping treatment personnel to better understand important personality characteristics that are directly related to response to a medical treatment environment, such as an interdisciplinary pain management program.

The Millon Behavioral Medicine Diagnostic

As an extension to the MBHI, Millon and colleagues subsequently developed the Millon Behavioral Medicine Diagnostic (MBMD). They did this because several important psychosocial characteristics were not evaluated by the MBHI (Bockian, Meager, & Millon, 2000). These include the following:

- Information concerning the presence of psychiatric indicators, such as anxiety and emotional stability, that could potentially influence patients' adjustment to their medical condition;
- Information on coping styles that reflect potential personality disorders;
- Information about other psychosocial variables related to cognitive appraisals (e.g., self-esteem, functional efficacy), resources (spiritual and religious), and contextual factors (functional abilities);
- Information about specific lifestyle behaviors (e.g., alcohol and substance abuse, smoking, exercise routine, eating patterns);
- Information about a patient's communication styles (e.g., tendencies toward disclosure, social desirability, preference for more or fewer details concerning medical information); and
- More detailed information that is useful for predicting patient compliance to a recommended treatment regimen, potential medication abuses, and emotional responses to stressful medical procedures (which, in turn, can be useful in health care management decision making and the triage process for mental health treatment).

THE STEPWISE APPROACH TO ASSESSMENT: AN EXAMPLE

I now present a brief example of the stepwise approach, using a patient who is referred for treatment of low back pain as an example (Figure 4.2). This has been presented elsewhere (Gatchel, 2001). Initially, of course, a comprehensive physical examination should be conducted with all patients reporting pain. This is part of the Agency for Health Care Policy and Research guidelines. This examination should consist of assessment and documentation of the following:

- range of motion, including lumbar flexion, extension, and lateral bend;
- straight leg raising;
- areas of tenderness;
- neurological signs;
- gait and posture (e.g., stiff, stooped); and
- Waddell nonorganic signs.

This examination will provide valuable initial information concerning possible functional limitations and anatomical/neurological problems. If needed, additional diagnostics can then be ordered. Also, signs of potential neuromuscular inhibition and motivational problems should become apparent during this physical evaluation, which can be further validated with information garnered from psychosocial assessment data.

Once it is decided that this low back pain patient can be safely functionally tested, a more comprehensive *functional capacity evaluation* should be requested in order to obtain the baseline data needed to individually tailor a physical rehabilitation program for that patient. This functional capacity evaluation should include the following:

- dual inclinometer range of motion;
- isometric muscle strength testing, including trunk extension and torso rotation;
- lifting capacity (isometric, isokinetic, and/or isoinertial); and
- cardiovascular and upper body endurance.

Additional functional activities tests, such as position tolerance, pushing/ pulling, and carrying, may be added to address specific work capacities.

In terms of the ideal approach for the assessment of possible psychosocial problems/issues in a patient with low back pain, Figure 4.2 also integrates the flowchart for the stepwise process introduced earlier, in Figure 4.1. The initial screening process to flag obvious psychosocial distress, which can be done efficiently, would consist of the administration of the BDI–II, the SCL-90-R, the Oswestry Low Back Pain Disability Questionnaire (Fairbank,

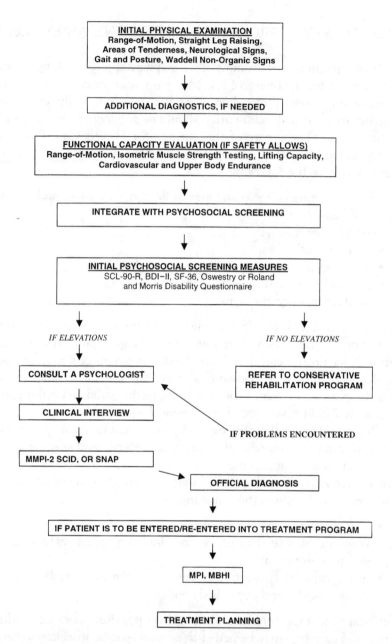

INITIAL PHYSICAL EXAMINATION
Range-of-Motion, Straight Leg Raising,
Areas of Tenderness, Neurological Signs,
Gait and Posture, Waddell Non-Organic Signs

↓

ADDITIONAL DIAGNOSTICS, IF NEEDED

↓

FUNCTIONAL CAPACITY EVALUATION (IF SAFETY ALLOWS)
Range-of-Motion, Isometric Muscle Strength Testing, Lifting Capacity,
Cardiovascular and Upper Body Endurance

↓

INTEGRATE WITH PSYCHOSOCIAL SCREENING

↓

INITIAL PSYCHOSOCIAL SCREENING MEASURES
SCL-90-R, BDI–II, SF-36, Oswestry or Roland
and Morris Disability Questionnaire

IF ELEVATIONS / *IF NO ELEVATIONS*

CONSULT A PSYCHOLOGIST / REFER TO CONSERVATIVE REHABILITATION PROGRAM

↓

CLINICAL INTERVIEW

IF PROBLEMS ENCOUNTERED

↓

MMPI-2 SCID, OR SNAP → OFFICIAL DIAGNOSIS

↓

IF PATIENT IS TO BE ENTERED/RE-ENTERED INTO TREATMENT PROGRAM

↓

MPI, MBHI

↓

TREATMENT PLANNING

Figure 4.2. The stepwise approach to the biopsychosocial assessment of a patient with low back pain. SCL-90-R = Symptom Checklist–90–Revised; BDI–II = Beck Depression Inventory—II; SF-36 = Short Form–36; MMPI–2 = Minnesota Multiphasic Personality Inventory—2; SCID = Structured Clinical Interview for *DSM* Diagnoses; SNAP = Schedule for Nonadaptive and Adaptive Personality; MPI = Multidimensional Pain Inventory; MBHI = Millon Behavioral Health Inventory. From *A Compendium of Outcome Instruments for Assessment and Research of Spinal Disorders* (p. 4), by R. J. Gatchel, 2001, La Grange, IL: North American Spine Society. Copyright 2001 by the North American Spine Society. Reprinted with permission.

Couper, Davies, & O'Brien, 1980) or the Roland and Morris Disability Questionnaire for Chronic Low Back Pain, and the SF-36. Pronounced scale deviations on these instruments would then alert the clinical staff to the degree of emotional distress or dysfunction in a particular patient and would indicate the need for a more thorough evaluation and a consultation with a psychologist. The psychologist's first step would then be the administration of a psychosocial clinical interview, reviewed earlier.

If there were no pronounced elevations displayed on the BDI–II, SCL-90-R, SF-36, and the Oswestry or Roland and Morris questionnaires, the patient can be referred directly into a conservative rehabilitation program. If the patient does well in the program, then no additional psychosocial testing is usually needed. However, if the patient does not do well, and there are problems noted by the staff (such as compliance, motivation, or fear of injury), then the patient will need to be referred to a psychologist for the appropriate consultation delineated above.

With both sets of physical and psychosocial data, the clinician can estimate the potential for getting the patient to change his or her behavior and work toward rehabilitation. Finally, with this clinical assessment material in hand, if it is decided that the patient is a suitable candidate to enter or re-enter treatment, an additional set of assessment instruments can be administered: the MPI and the MBHI. As I have discussed, these two instruments are beneficial for treatment personnel, who can use the results to identify the best approach for treatment management and to anticipate potential problems in the treatment program. In chapter 6, I discuss how the assessment material is used in developing a treatment program.

SUMMARY

Careful patient assessment is essential before any attempt is made to develop a pain management intervention strategy. The initial assessment process also provides the opportunity to start educating patients about pain mechanisms. This assessment should proceed from a global biopsychosocial diagnosis of pain to a more detailed evaluation of the most important interactive factors of this diagnosis. Using such a *stepwise* approach avoids the assumption that there is a single instrument that can serve as the best assessment measure. Indeed, several assessments will be needed. As was discussed, rather than asking which instrument should be used, a better question is: "What sequence of testing should I consider to develop the best understanding of potential biopsychosocial problems that might be encountered with this patient?" Of course, this stepwise assessment approach is only the first stage in the comprehensive assessment–treatment process. Once the assessment is completed, then it can be used in developing a treatment program individually tailored for each patient. In the next chapter, I discuss a comprehensive review of possible treatment strategies, and in chapter 6, I provide examples of integrating assessment and treatment.

REFERENCES

American Psychiatric Association. (1994). *Diagnostic and statistical manual of mental disorders* (4th ed.). Washington, DC: Author.

Asmundson, G. J. G., Norton, G. R., & Alterdings, M. D. (1997). Fear and avoidance in dysfunctional chronic back pain patients. *Pain, 69,* 231–236.

Beck, A., Brown, G., & Steer, R. (1996). *Beck Depression Inventory—II (BDI–II).* San Antonio, TX: The Psychological Corporation.

Bockian, N., Meager, S., & Millon, T. (2000). Assessing personality with The Millon Behavioral Health Inventory, The Millon Behavioral Medicine Diagnostic, and The Millon Clinical Multiaxial Inventory. In R. J. Gatchel & J. N. Weisberg (Eds.), *Personality characteristics of patients with pain* (pp. 61–88). Washington, DC: American Psychological Association.

Butcher, J. N., Dahlstrom, W. G., Graham, J. R., Tellegen, A., & Kaemmer, B. (1989). *Manual for administration and scoring of the MMPI–2.* Minneapolis, MN: University of Minnesota Press.

Clark, L. A. (1993). *Manual for the Schedule for Nonadaptive and Adaptive Personality.* Minneapolis, MN: University of Minnesota Press.

Cornwal, A., & Doncieri, D. C. (1988). The effect of experimentally induced anxiety on the experience of pressure pain. *Pain, 35,* 105–113.

Derogatis, L. (1994). *Symptom Checklist-90-R: Administration, scoring, and procedures manual.* Minneapolis, MN: National Computer Systems, Inc.

Dworkin, S. F., & LeResche, L. (1992). Research diagnostic criteria for temporomandibular disorders. *Journal of Craniomandibular Disorders: Facial & Oral Pain, 6,* 301–355.

Etscheidt, M. A., Steiger, H. G., & Braverman, B. (1995). Multidimensional pain inventory profile classifications and psychopathology. *Journal of Consulting and Clinical Psychology, 51,* 29–36.

Fairbank, J. C. T., Couper, J., Davies, J. B., & O'Brien, J. P. (1980). The Oswestry Low Back Pain Disability Questionnaire. *Physiotherapy, 66,* 271–273.

First, M. B., Spitzer, R. L., Gibbon, M., & Williams, J. B. Q. (1995). *Structured Clinical Interview for DSM–IV Axis I Disorders.* New York: New York State Psychiatric Institute.

Gatchel, R. J. (2000). How practitioners should evaluate personality to help manage patients with chronic pain. In R. J. Gatchel & J. N. Weisberg (Eds.), *Personality characteristics of patients with pain* (pp. 241–258). Washington, DC: American Psychological Association.

Gatchel, R. J. (2001). *A compendium of outcome instruments for assessment and research of spinal disorders*. LaGrange, IL: North American Spine Society.

Gatchel, R. J., Deckel, A. W., Weinberg, N., & Smith, J. E. (1985). The utility of the Millon Behavioral Health Inventory in the study of chronic headache. *Headache, 25*, 49–54.

Gatchel, R. J., Mayer, T. G., Capra, P., Diamond, P., & Barnett, J. (1986). Quantification of lumbar function, Part VI: The use of psychological measures in guiding physical functional restoration. *Spine, 11*, 36–42.

Gatchel, R. J., & Oordt, M. S. (2003). *Clinical health psychology and primary care: Practical advice and clinical guidance for successful collaboration*. Washington, DC: American Psychological Association.

Jensen, M. P. (1996). Enhancing motivation to change in pain treatment. In R. J. Gatchel & D. C. Turk (Eds.), *Psychological approaches to pain management: A practitioner's handbook* (pp. 78–111). New York: Guilford Press.

Kerns, R. D., Turk, D. C., & Rudy, T. E. (1985). The West Haven–Yale Multidimensional Pain Inventory. *Pain, 23*, 345–356.

Lasagna, L. (1960). Clinical measurement of pain. *Annals of the New York Academy of Sciences, 86*, 28–37.

Merskey, H., & Bogduk, N. (Eds.). (1994). IASP Task Force on Taxonomy. *Classification of chronic pain* (2nd ed., pp. 209–214). Seattle, WA: IASP Press.

Millon, T., Antoni, M., Millon, C., & Davis, R. (2003). *Millon Behavioral Medicine Diagnostic*. Minneapolis, MN: National Computer Systems.

Millon, T., Green, C. J., & Meagher, R. B. (1982). *Millon Behavioral Health Inventory* (3rd ed.). Minneapolis, MN: Interpretive Scoring System.

Roland, M., & Morris, R. (1983). A study of the natural history of back pain: Part I. Development of a reliable and sensitive measure of disability and low back pain. *Spine, 8*, 141–144.

Turk, D. C., & Melzack, R. (1992). *The handbook of pain assessment*. New York: Guilford Press.

Turk, D. C., & Melzack, R. (2001). *Handbook of pain assessment* (2nd ed.). New York: Guilford Press.

Turk, D. C., & Okifuji, A. (1998). Treatment of chronic pain patients: Clinical outcomes, cost-effectiveness, and cost–benefits of multidisciplinary pain centers. *Critical Reviews in Physical and Rehabilitation Medicine, 10*, 181–208).

Turk, D., & Rudy, T. (1988). Toward an empirically derived taxonomy of chronic pain patients: Integration of psychological assessment data. *Journal of Consulting and Clinical Psychology, 56*, 233–238.

Ware, J. E., Snow, K. K., Kosinski, M., & Gandek, B. (1993). *SF-36 Health Survey: Manual and interpretation guide*. Boston: The Health Institute, New England Medical Center.

Woessner, J. (2003, January/February). A conceptual model of pain: Treatment modalities. *Practical Pain Management*, 26–36.

APPENDIX 4.1

Recommended Readings

Gatchel, R. J. (2000). How practitioners should evaluate personality to help manage patients with chronic pain. In R. J. Gatchel & J. N. Weisberg (Eds.), *Personality characteristics of patients with pain* (pp. 241–258). Washington, DC: American Psychological Association.

Turk, D. C., & Melzack, R. (2001). *Handbook of pain assessment* (2nd ed.). New York: Guilford Press.

Woessner, J. (2002). A conceptual model of pain. *Practical Pain Management, 2,* 8–16.

APPENDIX 4.2

Back Pain

Common Reactions to Back Pain

Back pain is one of the most frequent problems seen by physicians. In fact, four out of five adults will experience an episode of back pain sometime during their life. Fortunately, the majority of back pain sufferers will successfully overcome their discomfort and return to normal social and work activities within 3 months, if treated appropriately. Of course, poorly managed back pain may cause medical complications and impair recovery. Moreover, there can be significant emotional suffering if it is untreated, undertreated, or inappropriately treated. For example, poorly controlled pain may lead to fear, anxiety, depression, and anger.

There are now some standard clinical guidelines that have been published for use in the primary care of patients, which involve symptom control when acute pain predominates (usually 0–10 weeks after injury occurrence). These guidelines emphasize the following:

- dealing with patients' fears and misconceptions about back pain;
- providing a confident explanation for the reason for the pain, as well as a prognosis; and
- empowering the patient to resume/restore normal activities of daily living through simple prescribed exercises and graded activity. This should be supplemented, when necessary, by adjunctive approaches, such as analgesics and manual therapy, for symptomatic relief.

Definition of Pain

It is quite normal to have certain emotional reactions to acute back pain, such as fear, anxiety, and worry about what the pain means, how long it will last, and how much it will interfere with activities of daily living. In fact, pain is a complex experience that includes both physical and psychological factors. Indeed, in 1979, the major professional organization specializing in pain—the International Association for the Study of Pain—introduced the most widely used definition of pain: *"an unpleasant sensory and emotional experience associated with actual or potential damage, or described in terms of such damage"* (Merskey & Bogduk, 1994, p. 209). As is evident in this definition, the emotional or psychological component is considered an integral component of the overall pain experience.

Questions You Need to Ask

With the above in mind, it is therefore important to ask your physician questions about the pain so that you do not leave the office still uncertain or anxious about it. Accurate information about your pain helps to decrease the anxiety it causes. It should also be kept in mind that, if your perception of pain exists beyond an approximately 2- to 4-month period (which is usually considered a normal healing time for most pain syndromes), then the pain begins to develop into a more chronic condition that may become associated with even greater psychological factors, such as heightened stress and feelings of helplessness. Indeed, during this period, feelings of helplessness, stress, and even anger toward the physician for not helping to decrease the pain, may occur. To help prevent the pain from becoming chronic, you need to be certain that your physician is attending to all of your important physical and psychological needs. The following should be addressed:

- Be certain that all of your worries about the pain symptoms are asked about and addressed by the physician.
- It is normal for patients to often fear serious disease or disability concerning the pain symptoms. Be certain that these fears are addressed by the physician through appropriate evaluation and tests.
- Be certain that your physician takes the opportunity to explain what was being looked for or ruled out during these evaluations and tests.
- If your physician recommends staying active, be certain that he or she tells you how to stay active safely.
- Be certain that your physician spends time identifying any functional difficulties associated with the pain (e.g., bending problems, lifting problems), as well as the plans for overcoming

such difficulties. Also have your physician address any such difficulties that may be associated with performing work activities.

- Be certain that any diagnostic information provided to you is clear, such as what *improvement* means and when it can be expected.
- Be certain that your physician provides you with information about the natural progression of back pain and a realistic prognosis of it.
- Whenever any recommendations are made, be sure that the physician writes these down so you can remember them after leaving the office.

Relationship Between Stress and Pain

All of the above are intended to deal with the emotional concerns and stress most patients have when experiencing pain. If you are not satisfied with the treatment you are receiving, always consider getting a second opinion from another physician. Otherwise, the stress and uncertainties and helplessness you are feeling may make your pain symptoms even greater. We know that anxiety and stress can actually cause an increase in the perception of pain. Therefore, if you are anxious and uncertain about the meaning of the pain, you will be more prone to experience greater amounts of pain that might last for a greater period of time.

It is important to remember that there is a dynamic relationship between your psychological state (e.g., stress level) and your physical state (e.g., pain). Pain can cause stress, which causes more pain, which causes more stress, and so on. This vicious cycle, once it starts to occur, can then be very difficult to break. In fact, if your pain and stress levels persist for more than 4 months, then there is often a greater increase in emotional distress and pain, which can become more chronic in nature. Once pain becomes chronic, there is a great deal more emotional suffering, including loss of sleep, inability to work, as well as feeling irritable and helpless about what can be done and attempts to relieve the pain at any cost. This may lead to trying any medication that is available, or any type of pain intervention (such as injection procedures or even surgery) to eliminate the pain. Although such invasive approaches can be beneficial for some patients, they often can be avoided if the stress and pain are appropriately dealt with at an early point in time. Of course, sometimes there is an obvious physiological cause for the back pain, such as a ruptured disk, which requires immediate surgical intervention. However, often, back pain might be due just to some soft-tissue strain or sprain that does not require any type of major surgical intervention.

Effective Interventions for Back Pain

As a patient, you need to be proactive and not allow the naturally occurring feelings of anxiety and stress to cloud your judgment in terms of methods of pain relief. The key in managing back pain is to not let it progress to the chronic stage. Good patient care, which usually merely involves the physician taking steps to reassure the patient that the pain is only temporary, helps to relieve a great deal of the patient's anxieties and fears. This goes a long way to help prevent the patient from becoming overly preoccupied with the pain, and helps prevent premature catastrophizing about the symptoms. Also, fortunately, there are a number of psychological interventions that have been successfully used in the management of pain. These include stress management, relaxation training, biofeedback, hypnosis, and cognitive–behavioral therapy (which is a method to reduce feelings of doom and helplessness). There are also medications available to help deal with sleep problems, anxiety, and depression. Such comprehensive pain management programs, when integrated with your medical care, are quite successful. Your physician can refer you to such a program if it is deemed necessary. Participation in such a program does not mean the pain is all in your head. Remember, pain is a complex experience that includes a close interaction of physical and psychological factors.

Note. From *Compendium of Outcome Instruments for Assessment and Research of Spinal Disorders*, by R. J. Gatchel, 2001, LaGrange, IL: North American Spine Society. Copyright 2001 by North American Spine Society. Reprinted with permission.

APPENDIX 4.3A

Cleveland Clinic Psychological Screen for Interventional Pain Treatment

Name: _____ Clinic # _____ Date: _____

Adverse Indicators	YES	±	NO
Nonphysiologic exam/inconsistencies	❏	❏	❏
Somatization	❏	❏	❏
Inordinate dysfunction/regression	❏	❏	❏
Inappropriate affect for degree of dysfunction	❏	❏	❏
Disincentives for recovery	❏	❏	❏
Anger/blame/external locus of control	❏	❏	❏
Poor support/foster dysfunction	❏	❏	❏

Disabled spouse	❏	❏	❏
Addictive disorder, active	❏	❏	❏
Litigation for pain/suffering/future disability	❏	❏	❏
Pending disability claim	❏	❏	❏
Developmental Factors	❏	❏	❏
Neglect/abandonment/loss	❏	❏	❏
Abuse/molestation	❏	❏	❏
Excess responsibility	❏	❏	❏
Social/academic failure	❏	❏	❏
Truancy/arrests/military "busts"/sociopathy	❏	❏	❏
Prior poor compliance/health maintenance	❏	❏	❏
Medication noncompliance	❏	❏	❏
Patient noncompliance	❏	❏	❏
Smoke with asthma/chronic obstructive pulmonary disease	❏	❏	❏
Diabetic noncompliance	❏	❏	❏
Morbid obesity	❏	❏	❏
Indications for Prior Psychiatric Treatment	❏	❏	❏
Major depressive disorder, anxiety disorder	❏	❏	❏
Chemical dependence, active	❏	❏	❏
Other mental illness	❏	❏	❏
Favorable Indicators	❏	❏	❏
Incentives for recovery	❏	❏	❏
Compliance	❏	❏	❏
Job record	❏	❏	❏
Responsible vs. project	❏	❏	❏
Stable childhood, responsible behavior	❏	❏	❏
Mood appropriate to extent of dysfunction	❏	❏	❏
Healthy supports	❏	❏	❏

Note. From *Psychological Screen for Interventional Pain Treatment*, Cleveland, OH: The Cleveland Clinic Foundation.

APPENDIX 4.3B

Examples of Four Items From the Mini–Mental State Examination

1. Example of orientation to time question
   "What is the date?"
2. Example of registration question
   "Listen carefully. I am going to say three words. You say them back after I stop. Ready? Here they are:
   HOUSE (pause) . . . CAR (pause) . . . LAKE (pause). Now repeat those words back to me."
   (Repeat up to five times, but score only the first trial.)
3. Example of a naming question
   "What is this?" (Point to a pencil or pen.)
4. Example of a reading question
   "Please read this and do what it says." [Show examinee the words on the stimulus form.]
   "CLOSE YOUR EYES"

Note. Reproduced by special permission of the Publisher, Psychological Assessment Resources, Inc., from the Mini–Mental State Examination, by Marshal Folstein and Susan Folstein. Copyright 1975, 1998, 2001 by MiniMental, LLC. All rights reserved. Published 2001 by Psychological Assessment Resources, Inc. May not be reproduced in whole or in part in any form or by any means without written permission of Psychological Assessment Resources, Inc., 16204 North Florida Avenue, Lutz, FL 33549. The complete MMSE can be purchased from PAR, Inc., by calling (800) 331-8378 or (813) 968-3003.

5

THE STEP-CARE FRAMEWORK OF PAIN TREATMENT

The quest to understand and control pain has been a significant human pursuit since earliest recorded history.

—Turk (1996, p. *xi*)

It is fortunate that in recent years there has been an increase in efforts to develop effective pain management methods (Jenkner, 2002; Lebovits, 1979; Turk & Gatchel, 2002). Further developments and refinements will continue to occur as more is learned about biopsychosocial pain processes. For now, health care professionals have an armamentarium of techniques that can be used. For example, in chapter 3, I briefly reviewed the step-care framework for managing back pain, introduced by Von Korff (1999). This same framework can be used in dealing with pain symptoms in general. Again, there are three basic steps in this framework:

STEP 1

This is the lowest intensity of intervention (or *primary intervention*, as I discussed in chap. 3), which consists of addressing a patient's fear and avoidance beliefs about the pain through education, information, and advice about the importance of returning to activities of daily living as soon as possible. It is applied usually to acute cases of pain of limited severity. This level of intervention can usually be brief during the initial office visit. It may be all that is necessary for a great number of patients with nonpathological pain. Suggestions made by Williams (1996), and reviewed in chapter 3, regarding potentially important issues to consider when treating acute pain patients, should be followed.

STEP 2

Step 2 refers to the need for increased intensity of intervention and is reserved for patients who may continue to report pain 6 to 8 weeks following the onset of an episode and who demonstrate persistent limitations in activities of daily living (i.e., *secondary intervention*). It represents "reactivation" treatment administered to patients who do not improve after primary intervention at the acute stage. Interventions at this level might include a structured exercise program or additional cognitive–behavioral strategies to deal with patients' fears and to help them resume their usual work and recreational activities. At this step, an extended visit or multiple visits may be needed in order to improve outcomes for patients who need this level of intensity of care. Also, such interventions could be efficiently provided in a group format, with the assistance of health care providers from other disciplines, such as psychologists, physical therapists, health educators, or nurses.

STEP 3

For patients who fail to improve with either Step 1 or Step 2 interventions, who continue to experience significant disability, and are at risk for becoming permanently disabled, Step 3 interventions might be required. Intervention at this step (i.e., *tertiary intervention*) may be more costly and complex than Step 1 and 2 interventions because they require an interdisciplinary and intensive treatment approach. Possible psychiatric comorbidity (e.g., major depression, anxiety disorders, substance abuse disorders), as well as secondary-gain issues (e.g., relinquishing responsibilities at work, at home, and in social arenas), will need to be addressed. If these services cannot be provided in the primary-care setting, such patients may need to be referred to specialty services, preferably an interdisciplinary pain management center (Deschner & Polatin, 2000; Mayer & Polatin, 2000).

As Von Korff (1999) noted, this *step-care framework* does not need to be applied only in a progressive fashion. Many times, patients may come to the attention of the primary-care provider already in need of Step 3 intervention for an ongoing pain problem that has failed to resolve and that has resulted in significant physical limitations. In such cases, a stratified approach is recommended, in which steps can be skipped and a patient can be immediately matched to the level of care appropriate for his or her needs. Again, these three steps are the same as the primary-, secondary-, and tertiary-care distinctions made in chapter 3.

TAILORING TREATMENT FOR EACH PATIENT

Of course, the step-care framework provides a broad, overall approach to pain management. As I noted in chapters 1 and 2, the importance of treatment matching for each patient is now recognized. As noted earlier, health care professionals now have a broad range of pain management techniques in their treatment armamentarium. A brief catalog of them includes the following:

- pharmacotherapy;
- interventional injections;
- surgical techniques, including implantable spinal cord stimulators and intrathecal opioid pumps;
- physical modalities, including ultrasound, exercise, transcutaneous nerve stimulation, and hot/cold packs;
- cognitive–behavioral strategies, including coping skills, positive imagery, distraction, and so on;
- stress management, including relaxation and biofeedback;
- hypnosis;
- acupuncture;
- operant treatment strategies;
- interdisciplinary pain management;
- individual, group, and family therapies; and
- modeling and social support.

Turk and Gatchel (2002) provided a comprehensive practitioner's handbook of the major psychological approaches to pain management. Later in this chapter, I present a prototypical 12-week course of cognitive–behavioral therapy (CBT) for patients with pain, especially for patients whose pain is becoming chronic in nature. Some of the topics mentioned were reviewed in chapter 3 (relaxation training, gate-control theory, the stress–pain cycle, etc.). Morley, Eccleston, and Williams (1999), on the basis of their systematic review of the scientific literature and a meta-analysis of randomized controlled trials, found that CBT produced significantly greater changes in self-reported pain and cognitive coping, as well as reduced behavioral expressions of pain, relative to waiting list control patients and alternative-treatment control conditions. Some of the components of CBT include the following:

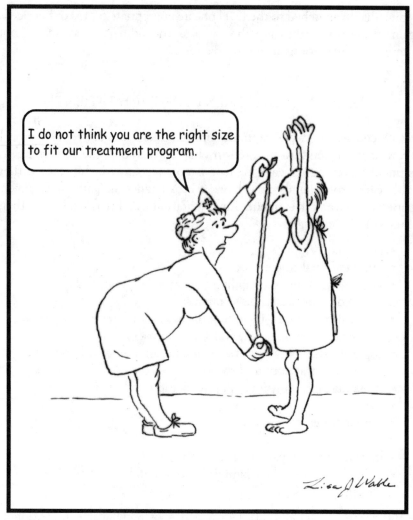

It is important to individually tailor treatment for each patient.
"One size or type does not fit all."

- educating patients about pain and their particular syndrome;
- helping patients to focus on increasing functioning and managing their pain rather than expecting a sudden cure;
- engendering a self-management and coping skills perspective to pain;
- providing coping skills in other areas, such as with interpersonal problems, marital problems, and so on;
- teaching relaxation and stress management techniques;

- emphasizing the identification and elimination of maladaptive thoughts;
- providing guidance about increasing activities of daily living, with appropriate pacing;
- providing ways to help improve their sleep;
- discussing the appropriate uses of adjunctive modalities, such as medications, exercise, and physical methods (such as heat and cold packs);
- assisting patients with appropriate goal setting; and
- providing relapse prevention strategies in order to help cope with potential future relapses.

Appendix 5.2B includes additional, more cognitively oriented coping skills methods for pain management.

A PROTOTYPICAL COURSE OF COGNITIVE–BEHAVIORAL THERAPY

Assessment

A multimodal assessment should occur before the patient starts treatment. An assessment should be conducted using a biopsychosocial approach in order to comprehensively understand the nature of the pain and the pain's impact on a patient's life. During the assessment process, it is also critical to explain to patients that you are interested in all the ways that pain has affected their lives and that you are not trying to prove that their pain is fake or that they are crazy for having pain that has not resolved.

Session 1

As with all CBT protocols, the first session is used to establish rapport and provide the rationale for the procedures to be used. Melzack and Wall's (1965) gate-control theory of pain is explained to the patient in understandable language as a rationale for developing coping procedures to manage their pain. Pain is described as a complex experience in which thoughts, feelings, and behaviors can all affect the perception of pain. An example may be helpful to use at this point. For instance, patients may be asked to think about a time when they stubbed their toe after a difficult day and then compare it to what it might have felt like if they had been at a party when they had stubbed their toe. Coping strategies are then described as learnable skills that the patient can develop as a means of closing the pain "gate." For instance, relaxation skills, cognitive restructuring, pleasant activity scheduling, and the practice of assertiveness skills are all things that can be taught. The steps that are needed to adopt new skills are described to the patient, including pinpointing the problem, gathering information about the procedure, discovering antecedents, discovering consequences, setting goals, contracting, and choosing rewards. The last thing that occurs in the session is instruction in diaphragmatic breathing and assignment of homework, including daily logs and material about managing pain. As with any CBT session, the end is spent making sure that all of the patient's questions have been answered and that he or she understands and can manage the homework.

Session 2

Each subsequent session begins with a review of the last session and a review of the homework. During the second session, a rationale for relaxation training is provided. The rationale includes a discussion of the physiological consequences of stress, individual differences in the ability to relax, and expectations for relaxation. With all of these techniques, self-efficacy is increased when the technique is framed as a skill that can be learned. The session is then reviewed for questions and concerns, and then an assignment (e.g., a pain diary) is given for the next session.

Session 3

This session begins with a review of the last session as well as of the homework. This session focuses on how to identify and incorporate relaxation training into everyday situations that produce stress. This process involves a review of the pain diary, which has been discussed earlier. Next, the patient is asked to schedule brief relaxation periods prior to those particularly stressful situations. Again, all sessions end with a review of the sessions for questions and concerns as well as the assignment of the next session's homework.

Session 4

This session begins with a review of the last session and homework, and then the rationale for distraction techniques is provided to the patient. Three distraction techniques are described: (a) focusing on physical surroundings, (b) counting backward slowly, and (c) focusing on auditory stimuli. An example of each technique is provided, and the patient is asked to practice.

Session 5

This session begins with a review of the last session and homework, and then the rationale for pleasant activity scheduling is provided to the patient. Examples are described to the patient, and possible barriers to engaging in the pleasant activity are reviewed.

Session 6

This session introduces the rationale for a pleasant activity scheduling plan. Step-by-step instructions are provided to the patient about scheduling pleasant activities. These include creating a balance between unpleasant and pleasant behaviors, planning ahead, setting specific goals, rewarding oneself for achieving goals, and checking one's progress towards one's overall goals.

Session 7

The rationale for cognitive therapy is provided in this session. Patients are taught about irrational negative thoughts. Homework is assigned to help patients recognize when they are having irrational, negative thoughts.

Session 8

Instructions are provided for changing irrational thoughts and self-instructional training. Patients are taught methods to change irrational thoughts, such as developing more rational alternative thoughts. The question "What evidence do you have for that?" is repeatedly posed to patients. Self-statements to deal with pain are also taught to the patient. Self-statements are broken down into four categories, including (a) preparing, (b) beginning, (c) during, and (d) after. These statements include "I may have to move a little slower, but I can still go shopping," or "My pain is flaring up, but it will soon pass."

Session 9

Methods for improving assertiveness are introduced in this session. A plan to improve social skills and assertiveness is developed with the patient; this includes developing a personal problem list, monitoring assertiveness, practicing with assertive imagery, transferring from imaginary to real life, and evaluating progress.

Session 10

The rationale is provided using a patient's newly developed social skills. Points that are stressed during this session often include the fact that it is important to have the opportunity to interact with other people and that inadequate reward occurs when social activities are no longer rewarding.

Session 11

Strategies for maintaining treatment gains are reviewed in this session. Points that are stressed during this session include: reviewing material already covered, reviewing what has been achieved, integrating what has been learned and incorporated into life, monitoring levels of pain and tension on a regular basis, and examining possible pitfalls and solutions to them.

Session 12

The major theme of this session is "making a life plan." Points that are stressed during this session include maintaining one's gains, planning effectively, and spelling out long-term goals.

THE POTENTIAL OF THE PLACEBO EFFECT

Before leaving this discussion of the step-care framework for managing pain, one should be aware of a potentially powerful adjuvant process for pain relief: the *placebo effect*. In brief, investigators such as Ader (2000) have broadly defined the placebo effect as a change in a patient's health status prompted by the positive emotional impact of a health care professional/healer or the healing environment. The placebo effect was originally shown to be an important factor in medical research when it was found that many times inert chemical drugs, which had no direct effect in physical events underlying various medical disorders, produced symptom reduction. There is an extensive literature on the placebo effect that undeniably demonstrates that a patient's *belief* that a prescribed medication is active, even if it is in fact chemically inert, often leads to significant symptom reduction (Shapiro, 1971). The placebo effect has also been found to be an active ingredient in psychotherapy and behavioral therapy, especially when anxiety is being treated (Shapiro, 1971). One important psychological factor contributing to the placebo effect that has been shown to affect the outcome of psychotherapy is the *generalized expectancy of improvement* (Wilkens, 1973). Thus, one can add to therapeutic effectiveness by strongly suggesting to patients that they will improve.

The placebo effect has also been shown to be involved in the reduction of pain (Baum, Gatchel, & Krantz, 1997). In a number of painful conditions, up to one third of individuals experiencing pain can obtain significant relief following the administration of a placebo (in the form of either a nonactive drug or a strong suggestion that increases a patient's expectancy of therapeutic improvement). The mechanisms involved in this placebo analgesia effect are still not totally understood, although factors affecting endogenous opioid activity appear important (Baum et al., 1997). Moreover, recent imaging studies of the brain are beginning to isolate other possible biological bases of the placebo effect (Mayberg et al., 2002). Regardless, though, it is clear that a clinician can help decrease pain in a certain percentage of patients by simply providing a placebo or a strong expectation of therapeutic improvement. Enthusiastic management of your patients' ability to manage their pain by following your therapeutic techniques goes a long way in maximizing the efficacy of those techniques.

SECONDARY-GAIN ISSUES

In the area of pain, issues of secondary gain have traditionally been viewed as major barriers to treatment and recovery, especially in patients with workers' compensation injuries. Disability behaviors are thought to be perpetuated by the perceived financial, vocational, and emotional awards that might arise from the psychosocial context of "being sick" for an extended period of time. Secondary gain associated with illness or injury was frequently and erroneously equated with conscious malingering, particularly when the potential for financial gain was apparent. However, as will be discussed, secondary-gain issues need not be major barriers to recovery in patients and can actually do a disservice to patients who may be erroneously labeled as unmotivated and resistant to treatment. As will also be reviewed, secondary-loss issues (such as financial loss, relationship loss, and the emotional consequences of loss) are also extremely important to consider in any pain management program.

What Is Secondary Gain?

Sigmund Freud originally introduced the concept of secondary gain, which he described as "interpersonal or social advantage obtained by the patient as a consequence of illness" (Freud, 1959). This should be differentiated from *primary gain*, which is conceptualized as an intrapsychic phenomenon by which anxiety is reduced through an unconscious defensive operation resulting in symptoms of a physical illness. Blindness, paralysis of a limb, or chronic pain for which a medical etiology cannot be isolated are examples of symptoms of illness perceived to be mediated by primary gain. Ultimately, the diagnoses of hysteria, a conversion disorder, or a nonorganic chronic pain syndrome were made in these patients.

As Leeman, Polatin, Gatchel, and Kishino (2000) reviewed, the basic concepts of primary and secondary gain were originally thought of as occurring along a continuum, in which secondary gain resulted from the symptoms initially created by primary-gain mechanisms. A patient's need to alleviate guilt or conflict was expressed in the physical symptoms (*primary gain*). A patient then was able to avoid certain activities in order to receive support from his or her environment that otherwise would not be forthcoming (*secondary gain*). Fishbain (1994) reviewed examples of secondary gain cited in the literature. They may range from the gratification of unspoken needs and wishes (e.g., to be dependent and taken care of, to take revenge, to change family dynamics) to more material concerns (e.g., financial gain, solicitation of drugs, avoiding sex, maintaining family and relationship dominance).

Secondary Gain and Treatment Outcomes

In recent years, the concept of secondary gain has taken on a life of its own outside the traditional psychoanalytic arena, especially in the area of pain management. Its association with an illness or injury is frequently and erroneously equated with conscious malingering, especially when the perceived scope of secondary gain is limited to financial issues (King, 1994). However, a much more enlightened view is that disability and abnormal illness behaviors will be stimulated by financial compensation according to basic principles of operant conditioning; that is to say, if patients are being paid to be sick, they will learn to continue those behaviors that reward them (Hammonds, Brena, & Unikel, 1978). This might lead to a simplistic explanation of cause and effect. Whatever the theoretical construct, one would assume that once the cause is eliminated, the effect disappears. Therefore, a common clinical assumption usually made is that once financial claims are successfully resolved, the alleged illness improves. However, researchers have not confirmed this but, rather have found that although exaggerated self-reported physical symptoms are more extreme when financial secondary gain exists (Rainville, Sobel, Hartigan, & Wright, 1997), favorable resolutions of financial claims do not necessarily resolve the perceived dysfunction or disability (Evans, 1992).

Many health care professionals have unfortunately made the assumption that patients with financial secondary gain issues are "untreatable" (Anderson, Cole, Gullickson, Hudgens, & Roberts, 1977). However, this assumption is seriously challenged by clinical studies demonstrating favorable treatment outcomes even in the presence of unresolved financial secondary-gain claims (e.g., Schofferman & Wasserman, 1994). One of the serious risks of an excessive focus on secondary gain is a premature and unjustified therapeutic discouragement, so that the clinician may rationalize a denial or lessening of care because the patient's prognosis is thought to be poor. As a consequence, surgery and conservative care may be restricted. None of this may ultimately be in the best interest of the patient (Gallagher, 1994).

Although a patient with financial secondary-gain issues overlying clinical complaints may be frustrating to the clinician, certain realities need to be recognized. First of all, in such a patient, self-heightened report measures of pain, suffering, disability, and emotional dysfunction (e.g., anxiety and depression) will probably be higher than in a patient with no secondary-gain issues, and these measures may not improve very much with treatment, even though functional measures do improve. Therefore, when treating such a patient the therapeutic focus should be on the correction of functional deficits and not necessarily on rendering the patient symptom free (Dworkin, Handlin, Richlin, Brand, & Vannucci, 1985). In fact, the clinician's orientation in such cases should be a biopsychosocial one, in which not only health issues are addressed but also labor market conditions, local economic characteristics, work environments, educational levels, household factors, and cultural values (Greenwood, 1984). To most effectively manage patients with pain as a major workers' compensation issue, it is important to have an understanding of the barriers to recovery that have the potential to delay clinical improvements and case resolution. Being sensitive to these barriers leads to a better understanding of a patient's motivation to change and to comply with a particular treatment or rehabilitation program. Treatment staff, case managers, and risk managers all may be more effective in their jobs and accomplish appropriate and compassionate case closure by comprehensively addressing these barriers to recovery. Disability behaviors are invariably perpetuated by perceived financial, vocational, and emotional rewards that arise from the psychosocial context of "being sick" for a long period of time. Changing these behaviors requires that these reinforcers be modified to encourage a more adaptive lifestyle. Techniques to accomplish this transcend conventional medical or psychological treatment. These techniques are discussed next.

Techniques for Managing Secondary-Gain Issues

When a patient has failed to respond as expected to a treatment regimen, that patient may need to be reevaluated from a biopsychosocial perspective to review all of the psychosocial, financial, occupational, family, educational, and cultural factors that may be influencing the expression of the pain and disability. After this reevaluation, the clinician will need to define a medical endpoint for the patient, even in the face of the patient's strong opposition. The clinician will need to organize all available medical, psychosocial, and vocational resources to implement a treatment plan that will be the final effort to resolve all pain disability issues and to return the patient to as normal a life as possible. Everyone who is involved in the patient's disability—family members, health care providers, insurance claims case managers, attorneys—may have to be enlisted to endorse this final rehabilitation effort to ensure its therapeutic success. Indeed, to manage secondary-gain issues, an assembled treatment team must accomplish the tasks listed in Exhibit 5.1. Leeman et al. (2000) discussed methods that can be used in realizing the goals listed in Exhibit 5.1.

In summary, the management of secondary gain in pain patients requires an awareness of biopsychosocial issues applicable to the particular case. Problematic and self-defeating behaviors can be controlled only when an overt dialogue has been established with patients for whom specific concerns are directly addressed by the treatment staff. This requires the health care practitioner to understand the educational, financial, and occupational expectations of patients and their families as well as the realities of the insurance system in which the injury or medical condition is being covered. Educating the patient about reasonable expectations may occur only after trust has been established. The health care practitioner must be a resource first, and an advocate thereafter, to help a patient resolve secondary-gain issues and effect a successful recovery and resumption of normal activities of daily living. Methods to deal with secondary-gain issues are reviewed further in the next chapter.

SECONDARY-LOSS ISSUES

Although the secondary-gain issues just discussed may be major barriers to recovery, a much larger barrier to effective treatment of pain patients may be the extensive personal losses that can arise as secondary features of chronic pain. Although the role of "secondary loss" in the well-being of the chronic-pain patient has not traditionally received significant attention among health care professionals, a new line of inquiry is emerging to examine its influence. As will be reviewed, secondary-loss issues are extremely important to consider in any pain management program. Losses, such as financial loss, relationship loss, and the emotional consequences of loss, can have a cascade effect, leading to increased emotional distress experienced by chronic-pain disability patients. Health care professionals unfortunately have traditionally ignored such loss issues. Any comprehensive treatment approach to pain disability, especially if it is chronic, will need to address such secondary-loss issues to maximize treatment gains. Once such issues are

EXHIBIT 5.1
Techniques for Managing Secondary Gain

1. Establish trust and rapport.
   a. Be the expert—become well versed in the jurisdictional aspects of the patient's case, and communicate this expertise in understandable terminology.
   b. Clearly communicate the goals of further treatment; success should be defined with improved function and return to as normal a life as possible (not as a cure).
   c. Be a source of logistical and social support.
   d. Be a patient advocate—for example, by providing clear documentation to assist the patient in resolving a claim.
   e. Demand something back—for example, compliance in treatment, pursuit of previously defined goals, acceptance of a medical endpoint.
2. Involve a disability case manager, that is, a trained medical professional who fully understands the vocational and disability aspects of medical illness.
3. Contain financial secondary gain.
   a. Follow the money and do the math—analyze current, potential, or perceived sources of disability-based income. This typically points to return to work as the better financial option and dispels illusions about a "pot of gold" at the end of the disability rainbow.
   b. Distinguish *impairment* from *disability*.
      i. A patient whose case falls under an impairment-based system (e.g., workers' compensation) needs to know that the monetary reward will have little to do with his or her functional abilities and pain and that, therefore, progress toward recovery will have no impact on the impairment assessment.
      ii. A patient whose case falls under a disability-based system (e.g., Social Security Disability Insurance) may be compensated differently depending on the type of job previously held and previous wages; in addition, professional opinions about work capacity, pain, and suffering may be taken into account. The patient needs to understand the previously mentioned treatment contract ("demand something back").
   c. Agree to provide medical documentation in exchange for patient's medical compliance.
   d. Discuss "pain behavior" talk—the patient must know that his or her pain level is being documented in the medical record and therefore the patient must eliminate exaggerated behaviors because they accomplish nothing and may be interpreted negatively as conscious symptom exaggeration and, therefore, malingering.
4. Incorporate vocational planning, which includes vocational exploration, deciding on a specific vocational plan, implementing this plan, and following up with the patient over the next 6 to 12 months.
5. Use multimodal disability management; an interdisciplinary treatment model is essential and must address psychosocial issues of importance to the patient (e.g., anxiety, depression, and anger; family issues; stress management).

Note. From "Managing Secondary Pain in Patients With Pain-Associated Disability," by G. Leeman, P. Polatin, R. Gatchel, and N. Kishino, 2000, *Journal of Workers Compensation, 9,* pp. 25–44. Copyright 2000 by Standard Publishing Corp. This material is used by permission of Standard Publishing Corp.

identified, the appropriate treatment within the context of a biopsychosocial program can be initiated.

Overview of the Concept of Loss

As Gatchel, Adams, Polatin, and Kishino (2002) noted, the experience of loss is universal to human life. Across a life span, individuals experience losses of many types and magnitudes, which can have a profound impact on their daily functioning, psychological well-being, and outlook on the world. Some losses may be restored, at least to some degree. For example, people can regain a lost sense of self-esteem, they can remarry after a divorce, and they can find employment after a job layoff. However, individuals differ from one another on how they cope with a loss, and some people are more affected than others by a loss. In addition, Rando (1988) suggested that the experience of loss can give rise to subsequent losses, compounding the complexity of the phenomenon and its impact on the individual's psychological well-being and functioning. Rando distinguished between a *primary loss*, which encompasses the initial event, and a *secondary loss*, which develops in the wake of the primary loss. For example, with the death of her husband, a widow experiences the primary loss of the spouse's presence. Subsequently, though, she also may experience secondary losses, such as financial decline, social isolation, and relocation of residence. The concept of secondary loss acknowledges that a major loss can have a long-term, rippling effect that reaches far beyond the initial event and that intensifies the trauma.

Individuals experiencing chronic pain and physical disability may be particularly vulnerable to the rippling effects of secondary loss. Indeed, anecdotal reports of personal loss among people suffering from chronic illness or pain have been extensively documented in the literature (e.g., Weiss & Weiss, 2001). These accounts suggest that loss events may infiltrate almost all domains of life, including physical functioning and autonomy, social relationships, financial stability, employment and familial roles, self-esteem, even a person's general worldview. Weiss and Weiss (2001) illustrated the complex loss experience that may accompany pain with their example of Lenny, a 43-year-old former truck driver who was unable to recover from physical pain and disability subsequent to an accident. In addition to the initial loss associated with the injury, Lenny went on to experience an overall reduction in the quality of life, including unemployment, increased stress in general and in familial relationships, a restriction of social contacts and recreational activities, and a diminished sense of identity and self-esteem. Lenny raised questions such as: "Who am I if I am no longer a provider, husband, father, friend, athlete, and man? What good am I if I can't do anything now?" (Weiss & Weiss, 2001). Indeed, when people go from being relatively autonomous to dependent, from vigorous health to chronic disability and fatigue, and from social engagement to isolation, it appears impossible for them not to feel cheated out of life and diminished as persons (e.g., Kelley, 1998). More broadly, they may develop an outlook on the world that is dominated by a sense of capriciousness and danger.

Employment Loss

For many patients struggling with pain, the loss of relationships is intimately tied to the loss of employment. For many disabled workers, the workplace represents their major social network and source of social support. Removal from the workplace because of disability results in a major structural and functional loss for these persons. Indeed, Price, Friedland, and Vinokur (1998) referred to job loss as a *network event*, which has implications that extend far beyond the individual. In addition to the experience of unemployment, job loss can produce a cascade of events that includes shrinking social contacts, financial strain, and familial stress as roles shift and change. An early work by Jahoda (1981) provides a very useful way of conceptualizing job-related losses. Jahoda distinguished between the *manifest functions* of employment, such as the capacity to earn money, and the *latent functions* of employment, including professional esteem, socialization, a sense of purpose, and a predictable and structured way to organize one's life's activities. Therefore, when a person experiences a job loss, the impact cuts across life's most vital aspects. The potentially far-reaching implications of job loss must be considered when one is assessing its impact on the disabled individual.

Emotional Consequences of Loss

The cascading losses that can occur with pain often exact a substantial emotional toll on its sufferers (Gatchel et al., 2002). Extensive research demonstrates that depression is a common affective correlate of chronic pain and that this population experiences more depression than do individuals without pain. In addition, a growing body of evidence suggests that anger has been underestimated for its role in the effect of distress on chronic-pain patients. Although most related research has focused on the connection of depression and anxiety to chronic pain, investigators are now recognizing the strong salience of anger and the emotional experience of pain patients, which can have a compounding effect on pain in the forms of dysfunction and diminished health (e.g., Fernandez & Turk, 1995). Such negative affective states can feed a destructive cycle in which the individual experiences increased problems and progressively loses coping abilities. One can view this negative spiral as similar to Seligman's (1975) concept of *learned helplessness*, in which the chronic-pain sufferer feels overwhelmed and ineffective in managing challenges, leading to exacerbation of depression, diminished coping, and an escalation of problems.

SUMMARY

In recent years, there has been an increase in efforts to develop effective pain management methods, resulting in an armamentarium of techniques that can be individually tailored for patients. As an overall framework to pain management, the step-care framework introduced by Von Korff (1999) can be used as a general template for dealing with the temporal stages of pain: *Step 1*, or *primary intervention*, applied usually to acute cases of pain of limited severity; *Step 2*, or *secondary intervention*, administered to patients who do not improve after primary intervention at the acute stage; and *Step 3*, or *tertiary intervention*, administered to patients who fail to improve with either Step 1 or Step 2 interventions. Within this broad framework, treatment matching for each patient can be accomplished with the broad range of pain management techniques at health care professionals' disposal. As well, clinicians also need to be aware of potentially important secondary-gain and secondary-loss issues in developing a treatment strategy. With these basic treatment guidelines, as well as the evaluation techniques reviewed in chapter 4, the health care professional is now ready to put all this assessment–treatment information together to implement the most comprehensive pain management program for individual patients. This is discussed in the next chapter.

REFERENCES

Ader, R. (2000). The placebo effect: If it's all in your head, does that mean you only think you feel better? *Advances in Mind–Body Medicine, 16,* 7–11.

Anderson, T., Cole, T., Gullickson, G., Hudgens, A., & Roberts, A. (1977). Behavioral modification of chronic pain: A treatment program by a multidisciplinary team. *Clinical Orthopedics and Related Research, 129,* 96–100.

Baum, A., Gatchel, R. J., & Krantz, D. S. (Eds.). (1997). *An introduction to health psychology* (3rd ed.). New York: McGraw-Hill.

Deschner, M., & Polatin, P. B. (2000). Interdisciplinary programs: Chronic pain management. In T. G. Mayer, R. J. Gatchel, & P. B. Polatin (Eds.), *Occupational musculoskeletal disorders: Function, outcomes and evidence* (pp. 629–637). Philadelphia: Lippincott, Williams & Wilkins.

Dworkin, R., Handlin, D., Richlin, D., Brand, L., & Vannucci, C. (1985). Unraveling the effects of compensation, litigation, and employment on treatment response in chronic pain. *Pain, 23,* 49–59.

Evans, R. (1992). Some observations on whiplash injuries. *Neurologic Clinics, 10,* 975–997.

Fernandez, E., & Turk, D. C. (1995). The scope and significance of anger in the experience of chronic pain. *Pain, 61,* 165–175.

Fishbain, D. A. (1994). Secondary gain concept: Definition problems and its abuse in medical practice. *APS Journal, 3,* 264–273.

Freud, S. (1959). *Introductory lectures on psychoanalysis, 1917* (Vol. 16). London: Hogarth Press.

Gallagher, R. (1994). Secondary gain in pain medicine—Let us stick with biobehavioral data. *APS Journal, 3,* 274–278.

Gatchel, R. J., Adams, L., Polatin, P. B., & Kishino, N. D. (2002). Secondary loss and pain-associated disability: Theoretical overview and treatment implications. *Journal of Occupational Rehabilitation, 12,* 99–110.

Gatchel, R. J., & Robinson, R. C. (2003). Pain management. In W. O'Donohue, J. E. Fisher, & S. C. Hayes (Eds.), *Cognitive behavior therapy: Applying empirically supported techniques in your practice* (pp. 273–279). New York: Wiley.

Greenwood, J. (1984). Intervention in work related disability: The need for an integrated approach. *Social Science Medicine, 19,* 595–601.

Hammonds, W., Brena, S., & Unikel, I. (1978). Compensation for work-related injuries and rehabilitation of patients with chronic pain. *Southern Medical Journal, 71,* 664–666.

Jahoda, M. (1981). Work, employment, and unemployment: Values, theories and approaches in social research. *American Psychologist, 36,* 184–191.

Jenkner, F. L. (2002). A global view of evolving pain treatment modalities: An historical perspective. *Practical Pain Management, 2,* 29–33.

Kelley, P. (1998). Loss experienced in chronic pain and illness. In J. Harvey (Ed.), *Perspectives on loss: A sourcebook* (pp. 183–204). Philadelphia: Brunner/Mazel.

King, S. (1994). Concept of secondary gain—How valid is it? *APS Journal, 3,* 279–281.

Lebovits, R. (1979). Loss, role change, and values. *Clinical Social Work Journal, 7,* 284–295.

Leeman, G., Polatin, P., Gatchel, R., & Kishino, N. (2000). Managing secondary gain in patients with pain-associated disability: A clinical perspective. *Journal of Workers Compensation, 9,* 25–44.

Mayberg, H. S., Silva, J. A., Brannan, S. K., Tekell, J. L., Mahurin, R. K., McGinnis, B. S., et al. (2002). The functional neuroanatomy of the placebo effect. *American Journal of Psychiatry, 159,* 728–737.

Mayer, T. G., & Polatin, P. B. (2000). Tertiary nonoperative interdisciplinary programs: The functional restoration variant of the outpatient chronic pain management program. In T. G. Mayer, R. J. Gatchel, & P. B. Polatin (Eds.), *Occupational musculoskeletal disorders: Function, outcomes and evidence* (pp. 639–649). Philadelphia: Lippincott, Williams & Wilkins.

Melzack, R., & Wall, P. D. (1965). Pain mechanisms: A new theory. *Science, 50,* 971–979.

Morley, S., Eccleston, C., & Williams, A. (1999). Systematic review and meta-analysis of randomized controlled trials of cognitive behavior therapy and behavior therapy for chronic pain in adults, excluding headache. *Pain, 80,* 1–13.

Price, R. H., Friedland, D. S., & Vinokur, A. (1998). Job loss: Hard times and eroded identity. In J. Harvey (Ed.), *Perspectives on loss: A sourcebook.* Philadelphia: Brunner/Mazel.

Rainville, J., Sobel, J., Hartigan, C., & Wright, A. (1997). The effect of compensation involvement of the reporting of pain and disability by patients referred for rehabilitation of chronic low back pain. *Spine, 22,* 2016–2024.

Rando, T. A. (1988). *Grieving: How to go on living when someone you love dies.* Lexington, MA: Lexington Books.

Schofferman, J., & Wasserman, S. (1994). Successful treatment of low back pain and neck pain after a motor vehicle accident despite litigation. *Spine, 19,* 1007–1010.

Seligman, M. E. P. (1975). *Helplessness: On depression, development and death.* San Francisco: Freeman.

Shapiro, A. K. (1971). Placebo effects in medicine, psychotherapy, and psychoanalysis. In A. E. Bergen & S. L. Garfield (Eds.), *Handbook of psychotherapy and behavior change* (pp. 439–473). New York: Wiley.

Turk, D. C. (1996). Biopsychosocial perspective on chronic pain. In R. J. Gatchel & D. C. Turk (Eds.), *Psychological approaches to pain management: A practitioner's handbook.* New York: Guilford Press.

Turk, D. C., & Gatchel, R. J. (Eds.). (2002). *Psychological approaches to pain management: A practitioner's handbook* (2nd ed.). New York: Guilford Press.

Von Korff, M. (1999). Pain management in primary care: An individualized stepped-care approach. In R. J. Gatchel & D. C. Turk (Eds.), *Psychosocial factors in pain: Critical perspectives* (pp. 360–373). New York: Guilford Press.

Weiss, B. W., & Weiss, L. (2001, November/December). Getting off the pain roller coaster: Identifying the psychological aspects of pain can lead patients on the right track to recovery. *Practical Pain Management,* 22–24.

Wilkens, W. (1973). Expectancy of therapeutic gain: An empirical and conceptual critique. *Journal of Consulting and Clinical Psychology, 40,* 69–77.

Williams, D. A. (1996). Acute pain management. In R. J. Gatchel & D. C. Turk (Eds.), *Psychological approaches to pain management: A practitioner's handbook* (pp. 55–77). New York: Guilford Press.

APPENDIX 5.1

Recommended Readings

Gatchel, R. J., Adams, L., Polatin, P. B., & Kishino, N. D. (2002). Secondary loss and pain-associated disability: Theoretical overview and treatment implications. *Journal of Occupational Rehabilitation, 12,* 99–110.

Jenkner, F. L. (2002). A global view of evolving pain treatment modalities: An historical perspective. *Practical Pain Management, 2,* 29–33.

Lebovits, A. H. (2003). Psychological interventions with pain patients: Evidence for their effectiveness. *Seminars in Pain Medicine, 1,* 43.

Lechnyr, R., & Lechnyr, T. (2003). Psychological dimension of pain management. *Practical Pain Management, 3,* 10–18.

Leeman, G., Polatin, P., Gatchel, R., & Kishino, N. (2000). Managing secondary gain in patients with pain-associated disability: A clinical perspective. *Journal of Workers Compensation, 9,* 25–44.

Turk, D. C., & Gatchel, R. J. (Eds.). (2002). *Psychological approaches to pain management: A practitioner's handbook* (2nd ed.). New York: Guilford Press.

Von Korff, M. (1999). Pain management in primary care: An individualized stepped-care approach. In R. J. Gatchel & D. C. Turk (Eds.), *Psychosocial factors in pain: Critical perspectives* (pp. 360–373). New York: Guilford Press.

Weiss, B. W., & Weiss, L. (2001, November/December). Getting off the pain roller coaster: Identifying the psychological aspects of pain can lead patients on the right track to recovery. *Practical Pain Management,* 22–24.

APPENDIX 5.2A

Cognitive Coping Skills Training Material

The materials in this appendix were adapted in part from the following sources:

Ellis, A., & Harper, R. A. (1973). *A guide to rational living.* North Hollywood, CA: Wilshire Book.

Kranzler, G. (1974). *You can change how you feel.* Eugene: University of Oregon Press.

Lewisohn, P. M., Antonuccio, D. L., Breckenridge, J. S., & Teri, L. (1984). *The Coping with Depression Course: A psychoeducational intervention for unipolar depression.* Eugene, OR: Castaba.

Lewisohn, P. M., Munoz, R. F., Youngren, M. A., & Zeiss, A. M. (1986). *Control your depression.* New York: Simon & Schuster.

APPENDIX 5.2B

Negative Thinking

People with pain may often have a number of negative thoughts and see the world through a type of a negative filter. We will learn to identify and change negative thoughts that may be causing unnecessary stress, tension, and pain in your life.

There is a direct connection between how you think and how you feel. It is not the events that cause you to feel stress and tension, but what you say to yourself about them.

- We are continuously taking in, and evaluating, information about the events occurring around us. These *automatic thoughts* occur when we react to a situation before we know that we have evaluated it.
- These thoughts, or *self-talk*, are not planned or intended; they occur quickly, and they may lead to inaccurate perceptions. Self-talk can occur in words, images, and memories, and it can directly influence how we feel.
- If you have ever found yourself in a situation in which you reacted very strongly and you weren't sure why, then you have experienced automatic thoughts. A good example can be seen in the way our parents can "push our buttons"; often we react without understanding why.
- Monitoring what you say to yourself about internal and external events (your self-talk) can be a powerful tool for changing the way you think.

It is important to understand that it is what you say to yourself about an event that creates your emotions and behavioral reactions to it. Often, people say, "Oh, my husband makes me so mad!", but actually every person creates their own feelings by choosing to react a certain way. If you create your feelings, then you also have control over them.

First, you need to identify beliefs and attitudes that may cause you to overreact. Many beliefs and attitudes have become such an ingrained part of ourselves and past experiences that we are no longer aware of them.

ABCD Model/Rational Self-Analysis

The ABCD model identifies beliefs and attitudes by analyzing our perception of events. The process occurs in four stages.

Stages

1. **A** is the activating event or stressor that initiates the process.
2. **B** is your belief system, including thoughts, attitudes, and beliefs associated with the activating event.
3. **C** is the behavioral or emotional consequences of the event, which are the feeling and actions that result from the activating event.
4. **D** provides the statements that dispute the negative thinking in **B**, by offering a rational alternative.

Assignment

- Continue to monitor your daily level of pain and tension using the Daily Log.
- Read the material provided in the following pages; use the worksheet "feelings" to identify the feelings of your self-talk. Then complete Sections A, B, and C of the Rational Self-Analysis forms each day, describing one unpleasant event or emotion that has occurred that day. Do not complete Section D at this time.

Thoughts to Consider

When completing the Rational Self-Analysis forms, for **A**, describe the event as specifically as possible. Watch for distortions of events based on your emotions. This will be important in identifying feelings. When completing these assignments, be honest—remember that you don't have to share them if you don't want to. You will benefit most from understanding how your negative thoughts are affecting your pain. Your understanding is the first step in changing your feelings and giving you more control over your life. Don't feel frustrated if you have problems at first; these techniques take time and practice. No one is content, completely stress free, or happy all the time. The idea is to keep negative feelings at a more manageable level so we can deal with life's difficulties more constructively.

- Many people who suffer from persistent pain have negative, self-defeating thoughts that can be damaging to their physical and emotional health. Ways we think can become automatic, with individuals not knowing how to break this cycle of negative thoughts and increased pain.
- We will learn problem-solving techniques that will help you discriminate between rational and irrational beliefs.

Feelings

Ten different types of self-talk are given below. Read each type of self-talk and identify how a person would feel if he or she used that self-talk.

B. Self-Talk	C. Feelings
1. I'm really good at putting things off, especially what I really don't want to do.	
2. So what am I going to do now?	
3. I must be a loser.	
4. I can't function very well with a cold.	
5. There must have been something more I could have done to help.	
6. She/he demands too much of my time and attention.	
7. I never get a day off and a chance to relax.	
8. Why can't they show some consideration once in a while?	
9. Stupid people; they should know better.	
10. It's not fair for them to talk about her like that; she really tries hard to be a good supervisor.	

Questions to Identify Your Self-Talk/Automatic Thoughts

- What was going through my mind just before I started to feel this way?
- What does this say about me if it is true?
- What does this mean about me, my life, and my future?
- What am I afraid might happen?
- What is the worst thing that could happen if it is true?
- What does this mean about how the other person feels/thinks about me?
- What does this mean about the other person(s) in general?
- What images or memories do I have in this situation?

APPENDIX 5.2C

Changing Negative Thoughts to Coping Thoughts

These are some thoughts that people with chronic pain sometimes report. Check the ones that apply to you, or write in some.

Negative Thoughts

There is no hope.
It is not fair.
I cannot go on like this.
I am a weak person.
I am useless.
I am worthless.
I can't do anything or go anywhere anymore.
No one understands my problem.
Nobody needs me.
I am not important.
Why me? I must have done something to deserve this.
I am a failure.
I am inadequate.
I can't take any more.
I am no longer attractive to my spouse.
If I can't enjoy myself, then no one should enjoy themselves.
I may get hurt if I try to do something for myself.
I have to depend on others.

_____
_____
_____

These thoughts can lead to emotions and feelings such as:
Sadness
Anger
Frustration
Guilty feelings
Resentment
Jealousy
Alienation, isolation
Fear

_____

_____

_____

One way to deal with these automatic negative thoughts is to try to change them to coping thoughts. For example:

Negative Thought	Coping Thought
1. I cannot do anything.	I may not be able to do everything I used to, but there are things I can do.
2. I am worthless.	I am not worthless; I still have value.
3. No one likes me anymore.	Some people may not like me, but some do.
4. There is no hope.	Change is possible—there is always hope.
5. No one needs me.	My family still needs me.
6. _____	_____
7. _____	_____
8. _____	_____

Disputing Your Negative Self-Talk

After one week of self-monitoring, you'll probably become more aware of the kinds of things you say to yourself at Point **B** that lead to the emotional overreaction you experience at Point **C**. Perhaps just becoming aware of some of your self-talk has helped you react differently to unpleasant situations or negative events in your day-to-day life. An additional helpful step is to dispute actively the things you say to yourself at Point **B**. By *disputing self-talk* we mean constructing arguments to use against your "should" and "ought" statements, against your beliefs that certain things are "awful" or "terrible," and against your overgeneralizations—the "always" and "never" statements. Some examples of disputing are provided below:

For "shoulds" and "oughts":	1. "Why should I or the other person behave in this particular way?" 2. "Why must an event occur just the way I wanted it to?"
For "terribles" and "awfuls":	1. "I would have liked this person to do or say this, but is there any good reason why they must say or do what I'd like?" 2. "I would have liked for this to have happened differently, but is it really terrible that they didn't do it?"
For overgeneralizations:	1. "Just because this didn't work out the way I wanted, is there any good evidence that it can't work out better another time?" 2. "Just because that person said something about me that I didn't like, does that really mean that everyone is going to feel that way?"

From now on, when you complete the Daily Log, be sure to complete Section **D.** For each of your negative/nonconstructive self-talk statements in Section **B,** in Section **D** write statements that dispute them or argue against them. As you complete Section **D,** follow our general guidelines, but use your own words to dispute self-talk. Review your past Daily Log sheets and complete Section **D** from all completed forms. From now on, complete all four sections for at least one situation each day: first Section **C,** then Section **A,** then Section **B,** and finally Section **D.**

You may soon notice that you are substituting constructive self-talk at Point **B** and that your emotional consequences are less stressful and/or take up less time. This is the goal for people using this approach. But don't worry if your progress seems slow at first. The self-talk most of us engage in at Point **B** has developed over a number of years and operates like an automatic habit. Like other habits that have bad consequences (e.g., smoking), it is not easy to change, and changing requires much effort and patience. Even if you realize that you have used negative self-talk only after you have reacted to a situation, there is still much to be gained from this experience. Analyze what happened, using the Daily Log. Try to identify the self-talk at Point **B** that caused your emotional upset at Point **C.** Then think of ways to dispute your nonconstructive self-talk. Next time, when that event or a similar one happens, you will be able to cope with it positively.

Also, keep in mind that nobody is happy, content, and stress free all the time. The goal is to help you cope when unpleasant events occur. We hope that by using this method, you will be able to keep negative feelings at a more manageable level so that you can deal with life's difficulties more constructively.

APPENDIX 5.2D

Thinking Errors

Thinking errors occur usually without our awareness, and they can cause us to distort situations and feel unnecessary bad feelings. Try to be open minded; listen to all thinking errors and see if you have ever experienced any of these either in yourself or in others.

All-or-nothing thinking occurs when you evaluate personal qualifications or situations in extreme, black-or-white categories. For example, before he developed chronic pain, a patient may have played baseball. Now he thinks to himself "If I can't play baseball, I can't enjoy any sport anymore."

- The advantage to thinking this way is that your life seems more predictable, more orderly, and gives you a sense of control.
- The disadvantage of this type of thinking is that our world is full of uncertainty, and living with uncertainty takes time and experience. The longer that you live accepting life's uncertainties, the more comfortable you are in it.

Overgeneralization happens when you interpret a single negative, such as a romantic rejection or getting fired from your job, as a never-ending pattern of failure that characterizes your life. People who overgeneralize the negative events that occur often feel hopeless and powerless to change the negative events in their lives.

- These were identified earlier in self-talk that uses words such as *always, every time,* or *never.*
- Remember that "misery loves company," and exaggerating your misfortunes will only make you and those around you feel worse.

Mental filtering is a tendency to pick out a single, negative detail and dwell on it exclusively, until you perceive the whole situation as negative. Individuals may focus more intently on negative aspects of an event or give more importance to the negative aspects. An example of this would be the following: You receive positive comments from most of your colleagues after your presentation, but one of them says something mildly critical. Then, you think about their reaction for days and ignore the positive comments.

Discounting the positive is the tendency to take neutral or positive experiences and turn them into negative ones. People can discount positive experiences by minimizing the importance or misinterpreting them to have a negative connotation. If you do a good job, you may insist that anyone could have done it, or that it wasn't good enough. This can make you feel unsatisfied, inadequate, and that your performance is never quite good enough.

Jumping to conclusions happens when we interpret a situation negatively, even though there is no evidence to support this conclusion. Jumping to conclusions can occur in one of two ways: mind reading and fortune telling.

- *Mind reading* is when you assume you know why someone else does what he or she does, without checking it out first. An example of this is the following: You say "Hi" to a coworker, and he does not respond. You think, "He must be made at me. I wonder what I did wrong?" When you ask the coworker, he explains that he was preoccupied with an argument he had earlier with his spouse.
- *Fortune telling* is a tendency to "know" that things are going to turn out badly. Based on your past experiences, you conclude this outcome as an established fact. An example is that you wake up late for work and get stuck in morning traffic. You say, "Now my whole day is ruined. I'll never get all the things done I need to do today."

Magnification occurs when you exaggerate the importance of a negative event. If you experience a flare-up in pain you may say to yourself, "I can't take this! I can't handle any more!" You may not want to handle the pain anymore, and that's okay, but you can stand it.

Minimization is when you do the opposite of magnification: You take personal qualities or events and reduce their importance until they seem insignificant or minimal.

Emotional reasoning is when you assume that reality is the same as your (negative) emotions. You believe that if you feel it, it must be true. An example is when you say to yourself, "I feel worthless." You conclude that you must be a worthless person, or you wouldn't feel that way.

Labeling is an extreme form of all-or-nothing thinking. This refers to identifying a mistake or negative quality and describing an entire situation or individual in terms of that situation. Instead of thinking that you made a mistake, you attach a negative label on yourself, such as "I am a loser/jerk/failure." For example, a person who suffers from chronic pain might say to herself, "I am defective and without redeeming qualities."

- Labeling a person is irrational; just because you do something that's stupid doesn't mean that you are stupid.
- You must have realistic expectations for yourself. You are only human, and humans make mistakes, and to expect yourself to never make any mistakes just doesn't make sense.

Personalization is when you take on responsibility for a negative event that is beyond your control. An example of this is a mother whose child is having problems in school. Instead of focusing on how to help her child change his problem behaviors, she feels that she must be a bad parent. She obsesses about what her child's behavior means to her and doesn't try to actually solve the problem.

Using *"should" statements* is when you tell yourself that things "should" or "shouldn't" be the way you hoped or expected them to be. They are attempts to motivate by guilt, yourself or others, into behaving in ways that you believe you should.

- "Should" statements directed against yourself can lead to feelings of frustration, guilt, anxiety or resentment. They also take away your direct control over a situation, as if you are complying with some external authority.
- "Should" statements directed at other people can lead to anger, frustration, or confusion. "Should" statements are negative thoughts that lead to feelings of frustration about things beyond your control.

Identifying Thinking Errors

I would like you to complete one entry on the worksheet labeled "Relating Automatic Thoughts to Primary Emotions." Look down the list of primary emotions and recall a recent situation in which you experienced one of these feelings.

- Describe the situation accurately, giving a good description of what was happening at the time.
- In the "Automatic Thoughts" category, list what you were thinking, your interpretation of the event, and what you were saying to yourself about it.

- Identify what thinking errors you were engaging in. Don't be worried if you find many of these thinking errors in your description of situations.
- Remember that identifying your thoughts is the first step to changing the way you feel.

Relating Automatic Thoughts to Primary Emotions

SITUATION	AUTOMATIC THOUGHTS	PRIMARY EMOTION	THINKING ERRORS
		SAD	
		FEAR/ ANXIOUS	
		ANGER	
		GUILT	
		LONELY	
		SHAME	
		HURT	

Note. From "Pain Management," by R. J. Gatchel and R. C. Robinson, in *Cognitive Behavior Therapy: Applying Empirically Supported Techniques in Your Practice* (pp. 273–279), edited by W. O'Donohue, J. E. Fisher, and S. C. Hayes, 2003, New York: Wiley. Copyright 2003 by Wiley. Reprinted with permission.

6

THE ASSESSMENT–TREATMENT PROCESS: PUTTING IT ALL TOGETHER

Art and science have their meeting point in method.
—Edward Bulwer-Lytton, British writer/philosopher

Now that we have discussed issues of pain evaluation and treatment, how can we put them into an overall gestalt in order to implement an integrated assessment–treatment plan? In this chapter, a number of vignettes are presented to illustrate such implementation. Other related issues that need to be concurrently considered also are highlighted.

STEP 1: BIOPSYCHOSOCIAL EVALUATION

As reviewed previously, the notion that there is a unique pain-prone personality characteristic is quite outdated. Some early works attempted to differentiate *functional pain* from *organic pain*. The term *psychogenic* was used to suggest that the pain was due to psychological causes only and that it was not "real" pain because a specific organic basis for it could not be found. This unfortunately significantly hindered the development of effective psychiatric and pain management strategies. Today, it is fortunate that the fourth edition of the American Psychiatric Association's (1994) *Diagnostic and Statistical Manual of Mental Disorders* does not list "psychogenic pain" as a diagnostic entity. The assessment or diagnosis of organically caused pain does not rule out the important role that psychosocial factors play for any particular patient. The general term *pain disorder* is now used, with subtypes coded according to the relative degree of psychological or medical conditions associated with it. Again, the biopsychosocial model now views disorders such as pain as the result of a complex and dynamic interaction among physiologic, psychologic, and social factors that perpetuates and may worsen the clinical presentation. The range of psychological, social, and economic factors can interact with physical pathology to modulate a patient's report of symptoms and subsequent pain and disability. The psychosocial concomitants of pain can be quite significant and are listed below. I discuss them in greater detail later in this chapter.

- *Psychological morbidity*: anxiety, anger, depression, suicide, sleep disturbances, somatization, substance abuse, loss of self-esteem.
- *Social consequences*: marital/family relations, intimacy/sexual activity, social isolation.
- *Quality of life*: decreased physical functioning, decreased ability to perform activities of daily living, decreased ability to work.

Therefore, one needs to conduct a comprehensive evaluation of both the psychosocial concomitants of pain and their potential interaction with the physiological concomitants of pain. As I reviewed in chapter 4, one must *not* make the assumption that there is a single instrument that can serve as the best assessment. For many patients, several assessments will be needed. As such, psychosocial/personality assessment should be viewed as a stepwise process, proceeding from global indexes of emotional distress and disturbance to more detailed evaluations of specific diagnoses of Axis I Clinical and Axis II Personality Disorders.

In addition to the above, and as I discuss in chapter 7, the determination of a patient's motivation for change is another important and unstated purpose of the interview process. Many patients with pain, especially if the pain is chronic, restrict their lives by avoiding any risk of experiencing pain, through immobilization and use of analgesics. Patients who are not candidates for intervention (for any reason), and who refuse to work toward active rehabilitation, clearly have suspect motivation for change. There are now methods for enhancing patient motivation in pain treatment programs (these are presented in chap. 7).

All of the above clinical information allows the clinician to contrast a patient's current psychosocial functioning with his or her past functioning and to compare the testing data with the interview data. The clinician can then estimate the potential for getting the patient to change his or her behavior and work toward rehabilitation. The domains that should be apparent to the clinician after careful evaluation are presented in Exhibit 6.1.

Finally, with this clinical assessment material in hand, if it is decided that the patient is a suitable candidate to enter a comprehensive pain

EXHIBIT 6.1
Domains of Which Clinicians Should Be Cognizant
After a Clinical Evaluation

- *Pain Experience.* The patient's subjective experience of pain, including ratings of pain intensity, frequency, duration, sensory qualities, and any associated disability.
- *Pain-Related Behavior.* Any overt behaviors associated with pain, such as bracing, grimacing, and so on.
- *Mood/Affect.* The effect of pain on the patient's affective state, such as anxiety, depression, anger, and so on.
- *Cognitive and Coping Skills.* Determination of the degree of current adaptive cognitive and behavioral coping strategies.
- *Social Functioning.* The impact of the pain on the patient's ability to engage and function in various social roles, such as work and activities of daily living.
- *Health Care System Utilization.* The over- or underutilization of health care facilities, including clinic visits, emergency room visits, surgeries, drug use, and so on.
- *Biological and Physical Fitness Factors.* The assessment of biological functioning, as well as the degree of physical fitness.

management program, an additional set of assessment instruments should be administered, such as the Multidimensional Pain Inventory (MPI; Kerns, Turk, & Rudy, 1985), the Millon Behavioral Health Inventory (MBHI; Millon, Green, & Meagher, 1982), and/or the Millon Behavioral Medicine Diagnostic (Millon et al., 2003), as presented in chapter 4. Of course, the thoroughness of this evaluation will depend on whether the pain is acute or chronic in nature. As I have emphasized, when pain becomes more chronic in nature, there are usually more significant psychiatric sequelae that develop. This is when psychopharmacological and cognitive–behavioral treatment approaches will need to be considered for possible use to address important psychosocial issues, such as pain-related depression, anxiety, and fear, as well as more pronounced psychopathology. As discussed throughout this book, the goal is to *manage* any pain or psychopathology in a comprehensive treatment program; attempts to cure psychopathology should not be the primary goal of a pain management program. In fact, clinical research has shown that, in spite of the degree of psychopathology, patients can successfully complete a pain management program such as functional restoration (Gatchel, Polatin, Mayer, & Garcy, 1994). Again, it is important for pain management personnel not to get trapped into trying to directly treat and cure psychopathology. Third-party payers will not reimburse strictly mental health services. One merely needs to appropriately manage the psychopathology in order to produce successful treatment outcomes. However, it is incumbent on the patient management team to refer out to appropriate mental health professionals whenever needed, after the comprehensive pain management program is completed by patients. A good referral-source list of mental health professionals in the community is a very important service to provide patients.

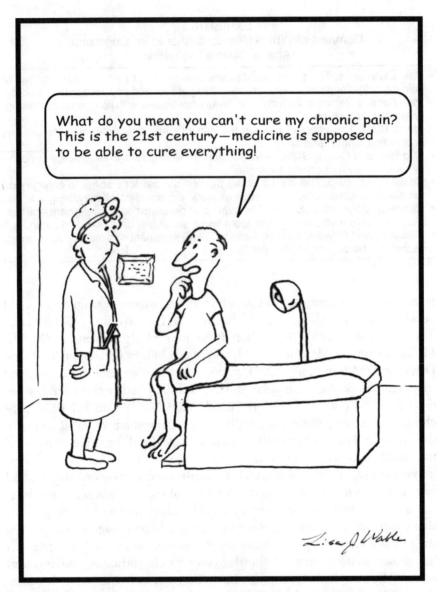

Most chronic medical illnesses such as hypertension, diabetes, asthma, and pain, cannot be cured but only managed.

Besides any significant psychopathology, there are usually some significant emotional components of pain that need attention in any comprehensive pain management program. This is because pain is ultimately a subjective, experiential state that involves a great number of affective properties. Turk and Monarch (2002) highlighted the most important of these affective factors. They are briefly reviewed below.

Depression

In an early study, Romano and Turner (1985) indicated that 40% to 50% of all chronic-pain patients experienced some form of depression. Usually, this depression is situational in nature, reflecting patients' reaction to their suffering with pain. Therefore, clinicians need to be ready to evaluate the possible presence of depression and its treatment.

Anxiety

Anxiety is also a very prevalent concomitant of pain, especially in chronic pain. Pain-related fear and concerns about avoiding additional harm and pain are quite common. Indeed, the threat of intense pain will capture the attention of anyone and is frequently difficult to disengage from. The constant vigilance in the monitoring of pain stimulation, and the often-misguided belief that it may signify a progression of a disease, can cause even low-intensity nociception or pain to become unbearable. As Turk and Monarch (2002) indicated, the fear of pain, which is driven by the anticipation of pain and not necessarily the sensory experience of pain, will prompt a great deal of avoidance behavior and retreat from normal functional activities. Such avoidance behavior is reinforced in the short term, because of the reduced suffering associated with nociception. However, such avoidance will eventually be quite maladaptive if it persists because it will lead to increased fear, limited activity, and other consequences that will significantly contribute to prolonged disability and persistence of pain. Indeed, some studies have demonstrated that fear of movement and fear of reinjury are better predictors of functional limitations than actual biomedical parameters (Vlaeyen, Kole-Snijders, Rooteveel, Rusesink, & Heuts, 1995).

Anger

There has been increased attention focused on anger as a commonly observed affective state in patients with chronic pain (e.g., Fernandez & Turk, 1995). Such anger may be precipitated by factors such as frustration associated with the persistence of symptoms and repeated treatment failures, anger toward employers and the workplace where the pain-related injury may have occurred, anger with insurance companies and the health care system in general because of the difficulty that is often encountered in trying to receive appropriate treatment, anger directed toward family members who are perceived as nonsympathetic, and so on. The negative consequences of such feelings of anger were pointed out by Kerns, Rosenberg, and Jacob (1994), who suggested that internalization of feelings of anger was strongly related to measures of pain intensity, reported frequency of pain behaviors such as grimacing and bracing, and perceived interference with activities of daily living. Although the precise mechanism by which anger and frustration exacerbate pain is not known, the role of heightened autonomic arousal has been implicated (Turk & Monarch, 2002).

Such feelings of anger are important to deal with because they may significantly interfere with motivation and acceptance of treatment goals and with the patient's forming a relationship with treatment personnel. Indeed, patients who are angry at the health care system in general, for example, will likely be less motivated to respond to recommendations from yet another health care professional at a pain management center.

Overall, besides the above emotional factors delineated by Turk and Monarch (2002), there are a number of other psychological factors known to influence the experience of pain. These include the following:

- uncertainty/ambiguity on the part of patients as to what to do,
- unpredictability of how long the symptoms may last,
- expectancy/anticipation factors as to what the best treatment will be,
- the meaning of the symptoms, and
- environmental factors that may influence pain symptoms (e.g., inadvertent reinforcement of pain symptoms by others).

The health care professional will need to address and deal with the above-listed factors during their initial contact with patients to reassure them and prevent unwanted contributions to pain enhancement. Also, compassionate patient care requires an understanding of some of the important losses that a patient has experienced. Such secondary losses were reviewed in the last chapter. Appendix 6.2 includes a more thorough discussion of the treatment implications of this issue.

STEP 2: BIOPSYCHOSOCIAL TREATMENT

With the above evaluation data in hand, the clinician can now tailor the most comprehensive pain management program for that particular patient. As has been reviewed, a number of important personality, emotional, and psychopathology issues can directly or indirectly affect a patient's report of pain and overall response to a pain management program. Thus, again, a biopsychosocial treatment approach emphasizes that a full range of psychosocial factors have to be addressed, in addition to any biological basis of symptoms. Interdisciplinary treatment focuses on providing patients with methods to better *manage* their pain, and the biopsychosocial concomitants of it, by providing an array of beneficial therapeutic modalities, ranging from physical therapy for reconditioning purposes; to psychopharmacological therapy to deal with emotional distress; to cognitive–behavioral therapy to deal with the affective, behavioral, and cognitive facets of the pain experience. Such a comprehensive treatment approach should result in significant changes in developing more appropriate beliefs about pain, better coping styles, and positive behavioral changes, as well as decreases in reported pain severity. It is important to increase function and perceptions of control over pain, because that will result in decreases in emotional distress and perceived pain severity ratings. Once again, to accomplish these treatment goals, it will be important to individually tailor treatment programs that are *matched* to a particular patient's biopsychosocial characteristics. This important treatment-matching approach was emphasized in earlier chapters. Health care professionals now fortunately have a broad range of pain management techniques in their treatment armamentarium to help tailor the specific treatment needs for each patient, after careful pretreatment assessment. These were discussed in chapter 5.

Finally, a major goal for many patients who have been disabled by pain is to get them back to work because of the many secondary losses associated with disability. To help these patients, a work transition program can be developed. For many patients, finding a job may be like "starting all over" in terms of job application skills. Appendix 6.3 presents examples of some of the skills a case manager may offer to such patients.

STEP 3: PUTTING IT ALL TOGETHER

I have discussed many issues concerning the assessment and treatment process. As I have emphasized, assessment and treatment must be carefully integrated in order to tailor an appropriate intervention program for a particular patient. I now present a number of cases to illustrate how this integration process is best accomplished. The presenting pain condition, as well as psychosocial issues often encountered with many pain patients, are highlighted for the various cases. Some of these cases were previously discussed by Polatin (1996).

A Neck-and-Shoulder-Pain Patient/Significant Somatic Complaints

A 50-year-old married woman was seeking treatment because of a recent "flare-up" of intense neck and shoulder pain, which had first occurred following an automobile accident 10 years earlier. There were no litigation issues outstanding on this case. The patient described her pain as "paralyzing" to her during the day, while doing housework. She also had a history of chronic headaches, as well as joint pain, which she attributed to arthritis. Her complaints of intense pain did not appear to be congruent with her actual observed movement and impairment during therapy. She regularly complained of pain but would often complete a required task, although it was a struggle and the therapist had to urge her on constantly. She would also often request rest breaks and passive means of pain relief (medication, massage, ice, etc.). (Polatin, 1996, pp. 318–319)

A medical evaluation of this patient revealed no active underlying pathophysiology associated with her pain. Initial psychosocial assessment with the Symptom Checklist–90–Revised (Derogatis, 1994) and the Beck Depression Inventory—II (BDI–II) revealed elevations in emotional distress and a moderate level of depression, respectively. As a consequence, the Minnesota Multiphasic Personality Inventory—2 (MMPI–2; Butcher et al., 1989) was administered to the patient. The MMPI–2 results revealed clinical elevations on Scales 1 and 3, suggesting some preoccupation with somatic complaints. During the subsequent clinical interview, the psychologist identified a number of issues.

- There were no apparent financial secondary-gain issues, such as personal injury litigation or workers' compensation issues. There were also no obvious other secondary-gain issues, such as avoiding household obligations.
- It was found out that the patient's husband had sustained a work-related back injury 6 months ago and has been disabled since. This had created some major stress because of financial problems. She indicated that she might need to return to work in order to earn more income. She was not very happy about this prospect.
- She reported that she has been feeling somewhat depressed lately and was not sleeping as well as she usually does.
- She presented to the interview well groomed and was oriented to time and place.
- In spite of her report of depression, she indicated that she had no current thoughts of suicide.
- An evaluation by a physical therapist indicated that she was becoming deconditioned because of her relatively sedentary lifestyle.
- She was very reluctant to discuss psychological issues, such as any possible feeling of anger toward her husband or anxiety about her present economic situation.

On the basis of the above biopsychosocial evaluation, as well as the chronic nature of the patient's pain, a Step 3 (or tertiary rehabilitation) program was recommended for this patient. Because it was decided that she would start treatment, the MPI was administered to evaluate her coping skills. The results revealed her to be an adaptive coper, which suggested that, with an appropriately tailored treatment program, she would have the adaptive resources to successfully complete it. After an interdisciplinary team staffing, the following treatment recommendations were made:

- The patient was placed on a regimen of amitriptyline (Elavil) to simultaneously deal with her moderate degree of depression as well as sleep difficulties. The medication level and symptom reductions would be followed during the next 2 weeks to evaluate the amitriptyline's effectiveness.
- A physical therapy program was prescribed for the patient in which physical reconditioning would commence with stretching and strengthening exercises that would be gradually increased in intensity. The physical therapist was advised to take a very supportive approach with the patient's pain complaints but to emphasize the importance of the physical conditioning and not allow the pain complaints to interfere with the progression.
- The patient was also prescribed a relaxation/biofeedback treatment regimen to help her deal with some of the anxiety and muscle tension that could be exacerbating her pain complaints.
- In addition, psychological counseling was provided to allow her to become more comfortable in discussing potential feelings of anger toward her husband's recent disability and the resulting greater demands placed on her, such as possibly needing to go back to work. During these sessions, she received instructions about the relationship between emotional distress and pain through basic didactics such as discussing the gate-control theory of pain and the pain–stress cycle.
- It was also recommended that she and her husband be seen in counseling in order to deal with any marital problems that may be related to his disability and her current pain complaints.
- Finally, it was suggested that vocational counseling would be available if she needed to return to work and help in finding an appropriate work situation.

This patient completed the rehabilitation program in 3 weeks, during which she reported a lessening in symptoms of depression as well as improved sleep. She actively participated in the physical rehabilitation program and reported that she felt much better because of it. The biofeedback and relaxation therapy was also found to be helpful in reducing the stress and tension, which, in turn, helped to decrease some of her pain. She now felt that, even though there was some small level of pain, she was better able to cope with the pain. During this time, her husband was still not able to go back to work, and she was required to find a job. She was fortunately able to find one without needing the help of a vocational counselor.

An Acute Low Back Pain Patient/Uncertainty About the Injury

A 30-year-old married man was referred by his primary-care physician because of a work-related acute low back pain injury that did not resolve 3 weeks after it occurred. The patient reported that he was very concerned about his ability to go back to work or whether his job would still be available when he became better. He was concerned about his family finances because of his inability to return to work. He had filed for workers' compensation, but only when his physician told him to because the back pain had not resolved. He felt confused and uncertain about what he should do, because this was his first such injury.

A medical evaluation indicated that the back pain was the result of a soft-tissue injury with no structural abnormalities. Because this was a first-time, very acute injury, the Short Form–36 (SF-36) was administered to gauge the degree of mental and physical health issues. The BDI–II was also administered to gauge the level of depression. The results from these tests revealed no clinically significant elevations, and a clinical interview was then conducted. During this interview, it was determined that this worker was very motivated to get back to work, and a major problem that appeared to be maintaining the back pain revolved around issues of anxiety and uncertainty concerning why his injury had not resolved and uncertainty concerning his future at the workplace. He had also been given very little instruction concerning what activities in which he should or should not engage, as well as the degree of bed rest he needed. He had also been prescribed a muscle relaxant medication that was causing him to be drowsy and inactive during the day.

With the above clinical evaluation data in hand, it was decided that a simple Step 1 level of care (or primary rehabilitation) was needed. Treatment was directed at providing reassurance concerning the short-term nature of this problem as well as specific instructions concerning physical rehabilitation prescribed by the physical therapist. The patient was taken off of the muscle relaxant medication and was put on a regimen of nonsteroidal anti-inflammatory medications. Treatment personnel met with him twice a week for the next 2 weeks to be certain that progress was being made. During this time, he was constantly reassured of the therapeutic improvement that he might expect. After 2 weeks, he was feeling much better and reconnected with his workplace to make plans to return.

A Work-Related Upper Extremity Injury Patient/High Degree of Reported Stress

A 45-year-old man presented with pain in the right upper extremity. He had been injured at work as a press operator when he sustained a crush injury to the index and middle fingers of the right hand. He was initially treated with reconstructive surgery to the hand, but thereafter his pain progressively increased, extending up the entire extremity into the neck. He subsequently had several decompressive procedures (including a right carpal tunnel release and a right cubital tunnel release), with some temporary relief of pain but recurrence within a period of 2 months and progressive worsening of the extremity pain. On presentation, he had almost no function of his right upper extremity, with some generalized wasting of the musculature and coolness and dryness of the limb. A diagnosis of reflex sympathetic dystrophy had been made. He had been referred for rehabilitation therapy in the past but had not been able to progress because of worsening of his pain. In addition, he reported that he had become more irritable at home and was fearful of harming his wife or one of his children because of temper outbursts. He had a very prominent sleep disturbance, admitted to feeling hopeless, and had thoughts of suicide. (Polatin, 1996, p. 323)

The initial psychosocial assessment of this patient demonstrated elevations on Scales 1, 2, 3, 4, 7, and 8 of the MMPI–2, and a score of 40 on the BDI–II, which put him in the high depressed range. The clinical interview subsequently revealed that the patient had been on military combat duty 20 years ago, during which he had witnessed a number of traumatic injuries and deaths. After his discharge and return to the United States, he received therapy at a Veterans Administration hospital for what was then diagnosed as a "stress disorder." Although he reported that he experienced improvement after a number of years, he still had occasional flashbacks and nightmares. In spite of this, though, he had been able to hold on to a job and lead a fairly normal life. However, these posttraumatic stress type symptoms had recently gotten worse after his current injury. It was also noted that he had extreme pain sensitivity, emotional lability, and insomnia, and he refused to use his right upper extremity because of fear of the pain.

With this clinical evaluation, it was decided to place this patient in an interdisciplinary functional restoration program (i.e., Step 3, or tertiary care). After the treatment staff reviewed all of the information about this patient, the following recommendations were made:

- The psychologist immediately initiated a nonsuicide agreement (i.e., the patient agreed not to attempt suicide) with the patient.

- Cognitive–behavioral therapy, with the training of coping strategies, was emphasized in order to deal with the recurrence of his posttraumatic stress syndrome symptoms as well as his emotional lability and distress.
- Relaxation and biofeedback training was prescribed to decrease his anxiety and emotional lability.
- Physical and occupational therapy was prescribed to deal with any job-related problems and decreases in physical functioning.
- Psychopharmacology was prescribed, placing the patient on a sedating antidepressant (Amoxapine), and clonazepam (Klonopin), which is a benzodiazepine and anticonvulsant, to deal with his high level of anxiety and emotional outbursts.
- Family therapy was also prescribed to deal with some of the irritability and problems experienced at home.
- Finally, group therapy was also recommended to provide some support with the biopsychosocial difficulties he was experiencing.

With the above program, the patient became much more emotionally stable, and his anxiety and depression levels decreased so that he was able to sleep better as well as function during the day more successfully. As he learned more appropriate coping skills, it was decided that he would be able to start thinking about returning to work. He then underwent vocational evaluation and was referred for job retraining after he completed the program.

A Neuropathic Pain Patient/Seeking a "Medical Cure"

A 55-year-old man was referred by his primary-care physician because of pain radiating down from his right buttock to his thigh and calf. He described the pain as "burning and shooting" down his leg. The pain had started about 3 months ago while he was on vacation, when he slipped and fell hard on his right side at poolside. He had a number of bruises and abrasions as a result of the fall, but radiographs revealed no bone fractures. The abrasions and bruises healed over a 2-week period, but the pain never abated. It actually had gotten somewhat worse, because anything touching that area, even the cloth of his trousers, produced an unpleasant sensation. He was having difficulty sleeping and concentrating on his work (he had a highly stressful job as an advertising executive), as well as a decrease in libido and overall energy level.

A comprehensive medical evaluation revealed no musculoskeletal or tissue damage to the areas associated with his pain. *Dysesthesia* (defined as abnormal, unpleasant, or unfamiliar sensations, such as burning, lacerating or burning pains, in the absence of any actual tissue damage) was noted, as well as *allodynia* (defined as stimuli that are nonpainful but nevertheless cause pain, such as any cloth touching his leg). Initial psychological testing with the SCL-90-R, the BDI–II, and then the MMPI-2, revealed that this patient had significantly elevated depression and anxiety levels. During the subsequent clinical interview, he had a tendency to minimize his mood disturbances and was much more concerned about finding a cure for the pain because of its functional and occupational limitations. With this clinical evaluation, and the difficulty often encountered in treating neuropathic pain, an interdisciplinary program (Step 3, or tertiary care) was prescribed. The therapist then outlined a comprehensive program for the patient, who appeared somewhat hesitant to engage in what he regarded as "non-medical" treatments. However, it was reviewed with him that biofeedback and stress management, as well as physical therapy, were important to help deal with the total medical illness he was experiencing. The MBHI was then administered to anticipate any potential barriers to effective treatment.

During the treatment team's review of this patient, a comprehensive treatment plan was recommended that included the following components:

- Initial biofeedback–stress management treatment was recommended to allow the patient to begin seeing the relationship between stress and his emotional distress. Once this was accomplished, cognitive–behavioral treatment would be introduced to help increase coping skills and address more directly his feelings of depression as well as potential self-worth and work-related issues.
- Amitriptyline (Elavil) was prescribed for his depression, because this medication also helps sleep as well as neuropathic pain (in a sense, it can be viewed as a "three for the price of one" drug). After appropriate titration, if there is not an adequate degree of pain relief, then Neurontin (an anticonvulsant) would be prescribed because of its positive impact on neuropathic pain. Because it has a sedating effect, it would be prescribed at night, to help the patient sleep. Finally, if depression is not being effectively dealt with by the Elavil, then a selective serotonin reuptake inhibitor, such as Zoloft, would be tried.
- A regimen of physical therapy was prescribed, after a physical therapy evaluation, because of early signs of physical deconditioning and the need to start mobilizing the patient.
- Group therapy was also recommended for its support benefits, as well as family therapy to use family members to reinforce positive active behaviors and to keep them involved in the treatment process.
- Finally, all treatment staff were instructed to keep track of any compliance issues and were advised that, many times,

neuropathic pain patients will initially have a pattern of "one step forward, and two steps back" before becoming fully invested and motivated in the overall treatment process.

After 3 weeks of treatment, this patient started to effectively use coping skills to more effectively manage his pain. He also came to realize that there was no magic "silver bullet" to cure his condition and that he would have to continue to use methods learned in treatment to adapt to the illness. He was scheduled for weekly booster sessions during the next month, until he was able to effectively manage his work stress. He was also referred out for therapy to deal with any unresolved work issues and the possibility of changing his career path.

The Failed Back Surgery Patient/Seeking a "Quick Fix" for Pain

A 65-year-old man presented to the clinic with complaints of low back and right leg pain. One year prior, he had had a surgical fusion of the lower back. Before this surgery, his primary complaint was of mechanical low back pain, which resulted in his inability to do activities of bending and lifting. He stated that the surgery did little help to relieve his back pain and, a few months after the surgery, he began to develop progressively greater right leg pain. The patient described his back pain as primarily constant, without significant aggravating factors. He also reported that his leg pain radiated from the right buttock down into the posterior thigh and calf and described it as burning in nature. When asked, he stated that the pain was evenly divided between his low back and leg. He had learned about implantable devices, such as morphine pumps, that were often found to be successful at reducing pain. He thought this would be a good option for him.

On a medical examination of the low back pain area, it was found that the surgical scar was well healed, but the patient had some muscle spasm and some abnormality in flexing and extending the back. The strength of the back was relatively normal, although a sensory examination revealed some loss of pinprick sensation in some areas of the back. Otherwise, the rest of the examination was unremarkable. X-rays of the lumbar spine revealed good fusion and no abnormal motion. During the psychological evaluation, in which the MMPI–2, BDI–II, and SF-36 were administered, it was revealed that the patient had a significant degree of depression and was experiencing a great deal of emotional distress. During the clinical interview, the patient reported that he had undergone multiple trials of nonsteroidal anti-inflammatory medication without any benefit. He was currently taking a narcotic (OxyContin) for the pain, but it was only partially effective, and he complained of side effects. The patient also indicated that he heard of new intrathecal opioid pumps that could be implanted to help with the constant pain and was hoping that he could receive one.

On the basis of the above biopsychosocial evaluation, it was decided that this patient would be best served in an interdisciplinary treatment program (Step 3, or tertiary care). The following recommendations were made:

- It should be consistently emphasized to the patient that interdisciplinary conservative care was the best option to relieve the pain that he was experiencing. A carefully prescribed physical therapy program was developed for any deconditioning problems being experienced by the patient. Occupational therapy was also prescribed to deal with any work-related functional deficits the patient might be experiencing.
- Cognitive–behavioral therapy was also prescribed to enhance the patient's coping skills to deal with the pain discomfort. In addition, a course of stress management/biofeedback was also instituted to deal with any muscle tension and anxiety being experienced by the patient. An antidepressant medication was also prescribed to deal with the patient's depression.
- It was also suggested that, if needed, some lumbar epidural or selected nerve root blocks might be beneficial. However, it was decided to forego such injection procedures until conservative care had a chance to produce some improvement.
- Group therapy was also prescribed to help this patient gain some support and education concerning the frequent "failed back surgery syndrome" that he was experiencing.
- It was emphasized to all staff members to not reinforce the patient's desire for an implantable device as a quick fix to this problem. It was felt that this may decrease the patient's motivation to work through the interdisciplinary program. However, it was indicated that if the patient did not show any substantial improvement in pain and functioning, then an implantable device might be considered. However, it would be provided only if the patient were deemed appropriate for it after undergoing a presurgical psychological evaluation (Block, Gatchel, Deardorff, & Guyer, 2003).

After a 3-week course of interdisciplinary care, the patient did start to demonstrate improvement in affect, pain relief, and functioning. It was decided to extend the treatment to at least another 3-week period to further reinforce the gains already experienced by this patient. At the same time, a return-to-work plan was initiated with the patient, and contact with his employer was made to transition him back to work.

Carpal Tunnel Syndrome Patient/Psychotic Symptomatology

A 32-year-old woman was referred for hand therapy 4 weeks after a right carpal tunnel release surgery. She had developed symptoms in her right wrist while at work as an assembler and was fearful that she would not be able to return to that job. She reported that the pain had not improved at all since surgery. She had been compliant with initial postsurgical treatment. She demonstrated residual tenderness over the operated wrist but no evidence of nerve compression; her pinch and grip strength were markedly decreased bilaterally. She attended therapy regularly, appeared compliant, and actually demonstrated gradual improvement, but she was still at suboptimal functional capacity after another 3 weeks of therapy. The pain complaint continued unchanged. She expressed discouragement and was noted to be tearful at times. (Polatin, 1996, p. 321)

Psychological testing indicated that this patient's MMPI–2 had elevations on Scales 1, 2, 3, and 5. She also had a high BDI–II score. During the clinical interview, she presented in an unkempt manner, and her mood was clearly anxious. She was time oriented but demonstrated some paranoid ideation and admitted to hearing voices. She reported that she felt safe at home and basically stayed in bed most of the day when she was not in therapy. During the interview, she also indicated that she had made a suicide attempt 5 years ago, which was followed by a 1-month hospitalization. At that time, she was put on an antidepressant and neuroleptic medication, which did help. Earlier, 12 years ago, she also had a brief hospitalization for psychosis but could not remember much about it. The initial medical evaluation also revealed that there was no longer any need for additional surgery.

On the basis of the above evaluation, it was decided that the patient be placed in a structured intervention setting, with Step 2 or Step 3 care as needed. The following recommendations were made at an interdisciplinary staff meeting:

- It was highlighted that attendance and compliance with any prescribed routines should be closely monitored by the psychologist, physical therapist, and occupational therapist.
- The psychologist should work with her in a supportive manner, encouraging her to acknowledge her depression as well as to understand that any hallucinations she experienced were related to the depression.
- She was also given coping skills training to deal with her current level of emotional distress and pain.
- An antidepressant, as well as a neuroleptic, were also prescribed to help her deal with her psychiatric symptoms.

During the course of treatment, the patient demonstrated an increase in positive affect and became less depressed. She began to work more easily in the rehabilitation setting, so that a vocational specialist was called in to meet with her employer to implement a return-to-work plan as well as any accommodations needed at work. It was recommended that, after she was discharged from the program, she continue in weekly psychotherapy for at least another 3 months, as well as receive medical supervision for any potential initial recurrence of her carpal tunnel symptomatology.

A Sickle Cell Anemia Patient/Adapting to a Lifetime Medical Illness

A 44-year-old woman sought treatment for whole-body pain stemming from a lifetime diagnosis of sickle cell anemia. Sickle cell anemia is a disease associated with abnormal hemoglobin molecules. As a result, the red blood cells become more fragile, leading to anemia, clogging of veins, and impairment of blood supply to many organs. The course of the disease is punctuated by crises of fever and episodes of pain radiating to the arms, legs, heart, and/or abdomen. This patient, when not in sickle cell crisis, experienced pain limited primarily to her lower extremities. She hoped that pain management treatment would allow her to reduce the frequency of crises requiring hospitalization and help her to manage her lower extremity pain.

At the time of the initial visit, the patient was taking hydrocodone, hydroxyurea (an experimental medicine), and folic acid. Her medical history was significant primarily for numerous hospitalizations over the course of her lifetime (beginning at age 4) for sickle cell crises and implantation of a MediPort. Her past psychological history was significant only for occasional trials of individual therapy for marriage issues and for job stress.

Psychological test findings (from the BDI–II, the Hamilton Psychiatric Rating Scale [Hamilton, 1960], and the MBHI) were consistent with mild levels of depression, with symptoms of sleep disturbance, hopelessness, sadness, decreased sense of worth, interest, and motivation, as well as decreased energy, indecisiveness, and attention and concentration difficulties. The results of the MMPI–2 also demonstrated probable fluctuating emotional states when under stress, increased physical focus, and negative self-appraisals of her ability to cope effectively with her current situation. During the clinical interview, it was also revealed that she was receiving disability income at the time of treatment initiation, which represented a significant loss of income for her family, as she had previously been the primary breadwinner. Although her husband worked, she had the larger income, stemming from her work as an advertising executive and writer for a major urban company. Her husband, a minister, had an inconsistent source of income and had to travel a great deal for work. On the basis of these clinical data, an interdisciplinary program (Step 3, tertiary care) was recommended.

After an interdisciplinary treatment staffing meeting, in which her case was presented and discussed with all team members, including the medical director (an anesthesiologist specializing in pain management), a physical therapist, and psychologist, the following treatment recommendations were made:

- It was recommended that, in addition to physical therapy, the patient would participate in 12 individual cognitive–behavioral health therapy sessions. The primary goals of therapy would be to teach her effective coping strategies for pain and pain-related stressors as well as to reduce depression.
- It was also recommended that she participate in 10 sessions of psychoeducational groups; physical therapy; and a visit with the clinic psychiatrist, who specializes in the unique aspects of pain-related depression. Soon after, she was started on Valium (2 mg), to be used as needed for agitation associated with pain and anxiety, which was identified by the treatment team. Later, the Valium was discontinued and the patient began Celexa with success.

Although the patient was very compliant with attendance to her sessions, she did have to cancel several sessions because of sickle cell hospitalizations. Consequently, she was seen over a 1-year period, with three additional booster sessions. A primary concern that became evident during the early phases of therapy was her perception of others' thoughts about the meaning of her pain. It was identified that her perception of others' doubts about her pain brought up painful childhood memories regarding her family's response to her pain. Her family reportedly communicated discontent and frustration about the pain-related intrusions on the family's otherwise healthy, normal lifestyle. By exploring these early memories and how they influenced her current experience and relationships with others, the patient was able to identify sources of cognitive distortions that were leading to increased current distress. Using a combination of cognitive techniques, such as journaling, maintenance of a daily log, and rational–emotive therapy, she was able to better understand her current emotional experience. This was then tied into education about the gate-control theory of pain, which helped her to understand the use of pain management techniques for both prevention of pain flares/sickle cell crises and a quicker resolution when already in crisis. Biofeedback therapy—specifically, temperature and respiration training—was also administered to assist her in applying relaxation techniques for both pain and stress management.

By the end of treatment, which was more supportive and explorative than the traditional pain management therapy conducted with musculoskeletal patients, the patient reported significant benefit. Specifically, she reported an increased ability to manage pain, a reduction in the frequency of hospitalizations, an ability to identify her role in the exacerbation/maintenance of family conflict, increased use of assertive skills, and increased coping abilities with both pain and emotional stressors. These gains were also reflected in repeat psychological testing, obtained at discharge. Her coping ability on the MPI changed from dysfunctional to adaptive, her pain level decreased, and her ability to manage pain (SF-36, Physical Component Scale [PCS]) decreased from a self-perception of severely impaired physical functioning to moderately impaired functioning. The patient herself was most pleased that she had also found a way to write about her pain and both address her previous writer's block and have a confidential outlet for her feelings about pain, the impact of pain on her life, and continued marriage difficulties. She was further referred for individual or family therapy in her area to address continued, long-standing marital difficulties.

This case again demonstrates the need for the practitioner involved in pain management to be flexible and creative in specifically tailoring a pain management program for each patient. There is no "cookbook approach" to all cases; the client's specific background and current circumstances need to be considered as well.

A Fibromyalgia Patient/Medication Detoxification Issues

A 58-year-old married woman was referred by her rheumatologist because of his concern about her escalating medication use over the past few months. She was diagnosed with fibromyalgia (a disorder characterized by multiple painful tender points/areas over the body [primarily above the waist], along with fatigue, dysphasia, irritability, and sleep problems). The symptoms first occurred approximately 3 years ago, soon after her last child had left home for college. She indicated that this "empty nest" syndrome played havoc with her emotions, and soon the fibromyalgia symptoms started. She got no relief from the constant low-grade pain after seeing multiple physicians, including her current rheumatologist.

A preliminary medical examination confirmed the symptoms documented by the referring rheumatologist. It was also determined that the patient was on a great many medications prescribed over the years by many different physicians (an antidepressant, an anxiolytic, a muscle relaxant, and medication for sleep, as well as multiple narcotic medications for pain). She was continuing to use all of them, as well as regularly using alcohol.

Because of the addictive nature of many of these medications, the high dosage levels being taken, and the patient's apparent dependence on them, a comprehensive psychological evaluation was conducted, including the MMPI–2, SF-36, BDI–II, MPI, and a clinical interview. This evaluation revealed that the patient was experiencing a great deal of emotional distress, as evidenced by multiple scale elevations on the MMPI–2, elevations on the physical and mental components scales of the SF-36, and a BDI–II score of 30. She also reported continuing problems with lethargy; sleep; pain; and a general feeling of being "scattered," which negatively affected her ability to concentrate. The Pain Medication Questionnaire (Adams et al., in press) also revealed a high rating for potential medication misuse.

On the basis of the above evaluation, it was decided that Step 1 treatment was initially needed for drug detoxification and stabilization purposes under careful medical supervision. Once this was successfully accomplished, a more comprehensive interdisciplinary pain management program (Step 3, or tertiary care) would then be initiated. At first, the patient denied the need for any drug detoxification. A meeting was then scheduled for her and her husband. This meeting focused on four major points:

1. When multiple medications are added over time, by different physicians, without careful coordination, there are often drug interactions that render some of the medications ineffective.
2. There are potential dangerous side effects and health risks posed by the long-term use of multiple medications.
3. The patient would not be able to start the interdisciplinary treatment program until after such detoxification, because the program requires taking control over all medications and eliminating other physicians from inadvertently negatively affecting treatment.
4. High-expectancy suggestions were introduced by relating to the couple the expected improvement the patient would experience if she were to complete the interdisciplinary program.

This meeting proved successful in motivating the patient to commit to the detoxification plan, with the support of her husband. It was decided to administer an outpatient detoxification program, because one of the treatment staff members was a psychiatrist with experience in such detoxification. It would also provide an early opportunity to confront any difficulties and resistance on the part of the patient before the start of the subsequent interdisciplinary program. The patient was asked to sign a medication agreement, and weekly meetings were scheduled for accomplishing the detoxification. Because this patient proved highly motivated, only 3 weeks were required for successful detoxification. It should be noted that less motivated patients require a much longer period of time (4–8 weeks). For some, inpatient detoxification may be required. Moreover, if a treatment staff member does not have experience in outpatient detoxification, then inpatient detoxification is the only alternative.

During the detoxification process, the patient was switched to a more effective medication regimen that initially included an antidepressant paroxetine (Paxil) and a nonsteroidal anti-inflammatory drug (NSAID) for soft-tissue pain. It was noted that if the antidepressant did not also improve the patient's sleep, then trazodone (Desyrel) might be added. Likewise, if the NSAID did not prove totally effective, then a muscle relaxant such as skelaxine might be added. Of course, careful titration to the most therapeutic dose level of all medications was monitored.

After stabilization on the new medication regimen, an interdisciplinary treatment program was tailored for the patient that included the following components:

- Stress management/biofeedback to help her develop some control over the somatic tension and anxiety she was experiencing. This was followed by cognitive–behavioral therapy to help her develop more effective coping skills to deal with her stress and pain. Issues relating to her empty-nest distress and feelings of abandonment were also addressed.
- Group therapy was also included to provide social support and a venue in which she could openly discuss some of her frustrations and life circumstances.
- Marital therapy sessions were also recommended in order to get her husband more involved in managing her illness behavior. A major reason for this recommendation was the fact that she voiced her anger toward his inattentiveness to her because of his busy business and travel schedule.
- Physical therapy was prescribed to deal with some of the major symptoms of deconditioning that were noted during an initial evaluation. It was emphasized that this therapy would have to be "ramped up" gradually to prevent any major flare-ups of pain complaints. Aerobic conditioning and pool therapy were considered the best initial modalities. Also, light massage was recommended to help with muscle tension and soreness.
- Continuing close monitoring/adjustment of medications was recommended.

After 3 weeks of treatment, the patient reported some major improvements. Her sleep had improved, and she felt less depressed and lethargic. She reported an improved ability to cope with the background pain, which was no longer interfering with her everyday activities. During the course of treatment, it was also discovered that she had retired as a schoolteacher after her children were born in order to pay total attention to them. She was counseled to consider re-engagement in at least part-time teaching to help fill the empty-nest void she was now experiencing. She subsequently acted on that recommendation and was making plans to apply for some teaching positions. She was also given information about fibromyalgia support groups in the area if she felt she needed any additional support in the future. Finally, she was seen in the clinic on a monthly basis during the next year for medication checks and relapse-prevention treatment.

A Skin Cancer Patient With Massive Facial Deformity/Death and Dying Issues

> A 66-year-old married man sought treatment for right-sided facial, neck, and shoulder pain, on referral from his otolaryngologist. His pain had begun 7 years earlier, after having been diagnosed with skin cancer occurring on the right side of his face. Consequently, he underwent a large number of surgeries on his face and throat, which were intended to contain the spread of the cancer and reconstruct his face and neck. However, these surgeries left him with horrible facial and neck disfigurement and essentially no oral cavity. He was thus unable to speak and used a marker board to communicate. He also underwent both chemotherapy and radiation. However, his pain continued to increase in spite of, and because of, his treatments.

During the medical evaluation, it was noted that his cancer-related pain occurred along with other medical conditions, including coronary artery disease, hypertension, emphysema, and rheumatoid arthritis. He also had a history of two myocardial infarctions and a stroke, and he had undergone a triple cardiac bypass, two hernia repairs, and cataract surgery on both eyes. He had not worked in several years, although previously he had worked in the construction trade.

At his initial behavioral medicine evaluation, it became quite clear that a major stressor involved a profound lack of spousal and family support. His relationship with his wife was contentious, and he saw her as fault-finding and argumentative. He felt that she had no sympathy for his pain and limitations. Psychological testing indicated that the patient was moderately depressed, though he initially denied the symptoms when asked (Hamilton Rating Scale for Depression and BDI–II). He suffered significant sleep disturbance, significant energy loss, and moderate psychomotor retardation. Testing with the MPI was consistent with his perception of others as punishing and unsupportive. Personality testing with both the MBHI and the MMPI–2 described a socially isolated individual who harbored significant feelings of bitterness toward others because of frequent perceived rejections. It characterized him as emotionally alienated, with underlying anger and depression and with very limited insight into his own emotional functioning. He was pessimistic, ruminative, chronically tense, and likely to experience his tension somatically.

After completion of his initial medical evaluation, a physical therapy assessment, and a behavioral medicine evaluation, the patient was discussed in an interdisciplinary staffing prior to initiating treatment (Step 3, or tertiary care). The following were recommended.

- It was decided that the patient would be offered four physical therapy and six individual behavioral medicine therapy sessions. The more typical series of 10 to 12 individual behavioral medicine sessions were not considered feasible with this patient because of his speech difficulties. However, if he benefited from the original course of six sessions, additional sessions could be considered.
- The main goals of therapy were to help the patient learn to cope more effectively with his facial pain while helping him to reduce his depression, anger, and feelings of alienation. It was also decided that he would forego participation in the educational groups because of his speech difficulties.
- The patient's medical treatment included prescriptions for a Fentenyl patch, Lortab elixir, Celebrex, and Neurontin for management of his pain. He reported some relief with these medications, yet his pain continued to increase. Consequently, his physician increased his medications with each follow-up visit. It became evident during the course of his treatment that his condition was likely to be terminal, because his cancer appeared to be spreading. Consequently, more of a palliative care approach was used in managing his medications, with the physician being less concerned about the possibility of his habituating to narcotic medications.

The patient attended his behavioral medicine sessions regularly. This was especially remarkable in light of the 2- to 3-hr travel time required for him to make his appointments (however, he was able to complete only five of the six scheduled sessions, because he was referred to hospice care before the last session could be completed). During the sessions, he communicated in a very cumbersome manner, using a dry erase marker board on which to scrawl his responses during the sessions. As a result, the pace of the sessions was quite slow, and his frustration at having to write his responses was evident. Nevertheless, he participated faithfully in every session. The first four sessions used the cognitive–behavioral techniques frequently used in this type of therapy. He was taught a series of stress management techniques to help him learn to reduce somatic stress levels. He was taught a meditation technique, a breathing relaxation exercise, and an imagery technique. Barriers to his practice of these techniques were discussed, which involved his rather uncooperative family members not allowing him uninterrupted time to practice the techniques. Problem solving this and other issues relating to his spouse and family conflicts was used. Educational issues relating to ways he could learn to manage his pain more effectively were also discussed. He seemed to be making some therapeutic progress, and he seemed to trust the therapist more than was initially the case.

However, as the sessions progressed, he reported progressively more pain, with pain medications becoming less effective in managing his pain, in spite of increased doses. It became increasingly clear that the customary cognitive–behavioral techniques were becoming less relevant for him because he was confronting existential issues concerning the likely terminal nature of his cancer. The cancer had begun spreading to his right ear and other areas, and he became increasingly pessimistic about the prospects of recovery. During the fifth and last session, the therapist again attempted to encourage the use of coping skills. However, it became clear that the patient was by now struggling with death and dying issues. Consequently, the therapist focused the majority of the last session on trying to help the patient face his death, which he knew was coming. No longer were they discussing ways of coping with his physical pain; now they were discussing the isolation he felt when no one would acknowledge his impending death. By responding to the immediate emotional needs of the patient, the therapist was able to make a strong connection with the patient and help him find some peace. His somatic stress and mild agitation were observed to decrease, and he was clearly engaged in the discussion, in spite of the cumbersome nature of his communication. He ended the session by indicating, tearfully, that the session had been very helpful.

The therapist subsequently learned that the patient had become too weak to make the trip for his last session. At about this time, his physician reluctantly discharged him early from the interdisciplinary program and referred him to hospice care in his own community.

SUMMARY

The theme of this chapter has been "putting it all together," to implement an integrated assessment–treatment plan. An initial comprehensive biopsychosocial evaluation, as reviewed in chapter 4, is first required. A number of important emotional issues often associated with pain need to be evaluated in order to develop a plan for best managing such issues. Depression, anxiety, and anger are common emotional factors associated with pain. With this careful evaluation data in hand, the clinician can now tailor the most comprehensive biopsychosocial pain management program for that particular patient. Many of the treatment approaches discussed in chapter 5 emphasized teaching patients how to better *manage* their pain and the biopsychosocial concomitants of it. Finally, a number of clinical vignettes were presented to illustrate how such an integrated biopsychosocial evaluation–treatment program can be successfully implemented. Of course, it should also be kept in mind that, regardless of the comprehensiveness and potential effectiveness of such an integrated assessment–treatment program, the patients' actual motivation for change is usually taken for granted. However, as I discuss in the next chapter, many patients need to be prodded, or motivated to play an active role in the assessment–treatment process. Without patient cooperation and motivation, even the best pain management program may be doomed to failure.

REFERENCES

Block, A. R., Gatchel, R. J., Deardorff, W., & Guyer, R. D. (2003). *The psychology of spine surgery*. Washington, DC: American Psychological Association.

Butcher, J. N., Dahlstrom, W. G., Graham, J. R., Tellegen, A., & Kraemmer, B. (1989). *Manual for the administration and scoring of the MMPI–2*. Minneapolis, MN: University of Minnesota Press.

Cohen, S., & Wills, T. (1985). Stress, social support, and the buffering hypothesis. *Psychological Bulletin, 98*, 310–357.

Derogatis, L. (1994). *Symptom Checklist–90–R: Administration, scoring, and procedure manual*. Minneapolis, MN: National Computer Systems.

Fernandez, E., & Turk, D. C. (1995). The scope and significance of anger in the experience of chronic pain. *Pain, 61*, 165–175.

Gatchel, R. J., Polatin, P. B., Mayer, T. G., & Garcy, P. D. (1994). Psychopathology and the rehabilitation of patients with chronic low back pain disability. *Archives of Physical Medicine & Rehabilitation, 75*, 666–670.

Hamilton, M. (1960). A rating scale for depression. *Journal of Neurology, Neurosurgery, and Psychiatry, 23*, 56–62.

Keefe, F. J., Beaupre, P. M., & Gil, K. M. (1996). Group therapy for patients with chronic pain. In R. J. Gatchel & D. C. Turk (Eds.), *Psychological approaches to pain management: A practitioner's handbook* (pp. 259–282). New York: Guilford Press.

Kerns, R. D., Rosenberg, R., & Jacob, M. C. (1994). Anger expression and chronic pain. *Journal of Behavioral Medicine, 17*, 57–68.

Kerns, R. D., Turk, D. C., & Rudy, T. E. (1985). The West Haven–Yale Multidimensional Pain Inventory. *Pain, 23*, 345–356.

Millon, T., Antoni, M., Millon, C., & Davis, R. (2003). *Millon Behavioral Medicine Diagnostic*. Minneapolis, MN: National Computer Systems.

Millon, T., Green, C. J., & Meagher, R. B. (1982). *Millon Behavioral Health Inventory* (3rd ed.). Minneapolis, MN: Interpretive Scoring System.

Polatin, P. B. (1996). Pharmacotherapy and psychological treatment. In R. J. Gatchel & D. C. Turk (Eds.), *Psychological approaches to pain management: A practitioner's handbook* (pp. 305–328). New York: Guilford Press.

Romano, J. M., & Turner, J. A. (1985). Chronic pain and depression: Does the evidence support a relationship? *Psychological Bulletin, 97*, 18–34.

Turk, D. C., & Monarch, E. S. (2002). Biopsychosocial perspective on chronic pain. In D. C. Turk & R. J. Gatchel (Eds.), *Psychological approaches to pain management: A practitioner's handbook* (2nd ed., pp. 3–29). New York: Guilford Press.

Vlaeyen, J. W. S., Kole-Snijders, J., Rooteveel, A., Rusesink, R., & Heuts, P. (1995). The role of fear of movement/(re)injury in pain disability. *Journal of Occupational Rehabilitation, 5*, 235–252.

Ware, J. E., Snow, K. K., Kosinski, M., & Gandek, B. (1993). *SF-36 Health Survey: Manual and interpretive guide*. Boston: The Health Institute, New England Medical Center.

APPENDIX 6.1

Recommended Readings

Block, A. R., Gatchel, R. J., Deardorff, W., & Guyer, R. D. (2003). *The psychology of spine surgery*. Washington, DC: American Psychological Association.

Fernandez, E., & Turk, D. C. (1995). The scope and significance of anger in the experience of chronic pain. *Pain, 61*, 165–175.

APPENDIX 6.2

Secondary Loss: Treatment Implications

A patient with pain is an individual who has usually sustained, at the very least, a significant primary loss (of good health and normal physical functioning), and consequent secondary losses that are determined by the psychosocial context of the pain and disability. As noted in chapter 5, common secondary losses include the following:

- economic loss;
- loss of meaningfully relating to society through work;
- loss of a social support network;
- loss of meaningful and enjoyable family roles and activities;
- loss of recreational activities;
- loss of respect from family and friends;
- negative sanctions from family;
- loss of community approval;
- loss of respect from those in helping professions (e.g., physicians);
- a new role that is not comfortable and not well defined;
- the social stigma of being chronically disabled;
- guilt over disability; and
- communications of distress, which become unclear.

It is strongly recommended that any comprehensive treatment approach needs to address such secondary-loss issues to maximize treatment gains. Once such issues are identified, then appropriate treatment within the context of interdisciplinary rehabilitation programs can be initiated. Indeed, early intervention with appropriate interdisciplinary treatment may help to circumvent the downward spiral of loss, psychosocial distress, and diminished coping. Such intervention may include the following:

- Depression is a known concomitant syndrome associated with chronic pain. As such, it demands prompt treatment, even independent of the chronic pain, with possible antidepressant medications and adjunctive cognitive–behavioral counseling and training.

- Group therapy and social support should be made available. Social support appears to be an important resource that can have a profound effect on the general well-being of an individual. Indeed, social support often can serve as a buffer or protection against the negative effects of stressful events and situations (Cohen & Wills, 1985). One important therapeutic modality that provides social support, as well as an environment in which secondary loss issues can be openly expressed, is group therapy. Keefe, Beaupre, and Gil (1996) comprehensively reviewed the role of group therapy for patients with chronic pain and found it to have significant clinical efficacy. Besides providing social support, such groups allow patients to deal with anger, emotional distress, and personal losses.
- Addressing pain and physical dysfunctions through physical and occupational therapies and accommodations will help patients become more active and to learn methods to reintegrate in the work environment and resume activities of daily living.
- Helping patients to apply for appropriate social and employment entitlements to help offset financial and physical losses is also very important. This is where a well-trained case manager can serve as an advocate for the patient in dealing with the often-myriad applications and forms needed to apply for short- or long-term disability and the consequent financial help that can be offered, as well as vocational retraining when appropriate.

Of course, each of the above cannot be used as the sole treatment modality for dealing with primary and secondary losses. Individual treatment may also be vital for patients who are especially overwhelmed by losses. Again, however, an integrated and comprehensive biopsychosocial treatment program is required. As discussed throughout this book, such a biopsychosocial approach will require specific assessment and therapeutic attention to the patient's experience of primary loss, one's belief system about his or her illness, current and prior coping abilities, and related secondary gains and losses. Once these perceived losses have been identified, they can be systematically addressed within the context of interdisciplinary treatment. Interventions might include treating biological depression, implementing effective medication and psychological controls for chronic pain, addressing family dysfunction, assisting in application to appropriate entitlements to counter financial and physical losses, facilitating grief counseling and adaptive readjustment to perceived losses, and correcting physical dysfunctions through physical/occupational therapies and accommodations.

APPENDIX 6.3A

Topics of Discussion Relating to Return-to-Work Issues

- What are your fears and anxieties about returning to work with same/different employers?
- What are you looking forward to?
- What would each of you like to take from our treatment program when you leave?
- What do you wish could have happened that did not, or could have, happened differently during our treatment program?
- Has your outlook on life changed since completing our treatment program?

APPENDIX 6.3B

Where to Look for Jobs

- Newspaper employment advertisements
- Word of mouth (friends or family members)
- Walk-ins (going in person to ask about potential openings and filling out applications)
- Going to your local state Workforce Commission and looking at openings (we can provide you with the location nearest to you). The state Workforce Commission, is a state agency that is available for everyone who is looking for a job to utilize. They have books with current jobs listings for all areas in the state, or they have this information compiled into a database that you can look up on their computers. Best of all, it's free. Each state has its own unique workforce commission.
- Looking on the Internet for job openings (if you do not have access to a computer, you can go to your local public library and use the Internet for free). On some sites, you can even post your resume for employers to see.

APPENDIX 6.3C

Internet Web Sites for Job Searches

- www.jobs.com
- www.monster.com

- www.dfwemployment.com
- www.careerbuilder.com
- www.hotjobs.com
- www.nationjobs.com
- Local job banks such as http://www.twc.state.tx.us/jobs/job. html (On this site, you can either click on the speed search or go down to the job seekers section and click on that.)
- http://stats.bls.gov/oco/ocoiab.htm (occupational outlook handbook) This site will let you look at different job titles and will give detailed information about each job, such as job outlook, general job descriptions, national average wages, and the educational/training requirements necessary to obtain the position and working conditions.
- Local newspapers (many newspapers now have their employment ads on the Internet)

APPENDIX 6.3D

Resume Worksheet

Objective Statement

"to obtain a challenging position as a/an _____ that will utilize my skills and experience." Be sure to list a specific occupation, such as: Administrative Assistant, Customer Service Representative, Welder, or a specific field (i.e., Customer Service, Office Setting, Manufacturing).

Skills

List 3–5 skills that you possess:

i.e., types 50 words per minute

Good organizational skills

Learns new concepts and techniques easily

5+ years experience as a computer programmer

Work Experience

List the company name followed by the city and state in which it was located

List your job title

List 3 to 4 job duties (depending on how much space you have and how many job duties you performed)

To the right or left of each employer, put the month and year you worked at each job.

> e.g., The Shoe Factory   Arlington, TX   5–99
>
> Sales Associate
> - Stocking merchandise
> - Assisting customers
> - Setting up displays

Education

List the names and city, state, degree/certification, and year graduated/completed.

> e.g., Arlington High School   Arlington, TX
>   High School Diploma   1994
>   or
>   University of Texas at Arlington   Arlington, TX
>   B.A. Business

Also include any training seminars, workshops, and other important educational information (i.e., CPR certification).

References

List 3 people who are:
- Not relatives (try to include one former boss/coworker)
- Willing to say good things about you

Also include:
- Name
- Title
- Address
- Phone number
- How you know them (friend, coworker, etc.)
- How long you have known them

III

SPECIAL ISSUES

7

MOTIVATION ISSUES

Researchers continue to try to discover the sources of motivation. . . .
Drives, incentives, needs, arousal, reinforcement . . . are viewed by
various researchers as sources of motivation.

—A. C. Parham (1983)

Despite the availability of effective pain management techniques, there remain many patients who do not improve or who actually relapse. Much of this failure can be traced to low patient motivation for treatment and its compliance requirements. Some of the reasons for potential motivation/ compliance issues, such as secondary-gain and secondary-loss factors, were discussed in chapters 5 and 6. Moreover, as I noted earlier (Gatchel, 1991), Pilowsky (1978b) originally formulated the concept of *abnormal illness behavior* as a method useful for understanding and treating patients with exaggerated physical symptoms or complaints that did not match the severity of any diagnosed pathophysiology. His formulation stemmed from earlier "sick role" (Parsons, 1964) and "illness behavior" (Pilowsky, 1978a) models that focused on aspects of behavior associated with being sick—that is, what people do when they are sick. The sick role has both advantages and disadvantages. On the one hand, sick people are sometimes stigmatized with all the attendant social awkwardness and decreased attractiveness that being sick entails. On the other hand, though, they are excused from their normal responsibilities and obligations. Indeed, some patients may be highly motivated to seek the protection that being sick entails, as a way of evading responsibilities and being exempted from social obligations. This may then become a potent reinforcer for not becoming "healthy." Treatment staff, therefore, must be alert to these potential barriers to recovery—whether psychological, legal, financial, familial, or job related—for remaining "sick." This knowledge allows treatment personnel not only to better understand and serve the patient but also to be more effective in problem solving when the patient is not therapeutically progressing as expected.

In this chapter, I review the important issue of motivation in pain management. M. P. Jensen, Nielson, and Kerns (2003) provided a comprehensive review of the motivational model of pain self-management, which is discussed in this chapter, that is helpful in conceptualizing how to deal with potential barriers to recovery. In addition, they provided a very cogent quote from Mark Twain that nicely summarizes what health care professionals often seemingly ask of their patients when attempting to motivate them to change (M. P. Jensen et al., 2003, p. 471): "The only way to keep your health is to eat what you don't want, drink what you don't like, and do what you'd rather not."

THE STAGES-OF-CHANGE MODEL

The *stages-of-change model*, introduced by Prochaska, DiClemente, and Norcross (1992), is a very helpful heuristic for conceptualizing patients' readiness to make necessary changes. DiClemente and Prochaska (1982) originally delineated specific stages through which individuals move as they change their maladaptive behaviors to adaptive ones. According to these investigators, people can vary in the degree to which they are ready to engage in new adaptive behaviors. Each stage poses unique challenges for the person that need to be addressed before that individual can move on to the next stage (Prochaska et al., 1992). There are six basic changes in this model:

1. The *precontemplation* stage is the one at which people are not even considering any changes in their behavior and may actually display active resistance to change if they feel they are being coerced into changing some behavior that other people view as a problem.
2. The *contemplation stage* is the point at which the individual now views the need for change and is starting to seriously consider making some change in the near future; however, he or she still has not yet committed to that change and is merely weighing the pros and cons of changing his or her behavior.
3. The *preparation/decision-making/determination stage* is the point at which an intention to make changes and initial behavioral steps in that direction of change are made.

4. The *action stage* is associated with concrete activities that will lead to the desired behavioral change.
5. The *maintenance stage* involves individuals making appropriate efforts to sustain the changes made during the previous (action) stage.
6. Individuals who are unable to sustain the changes they had made are viewed to be in the *relapse stage*. From this relapse stage, the individual may re-enter the change stage at any point (e.g., he or she might completely give up and go back to the precontemplation stage, or he or she may start right back again at the action stage).

With this stages-of-change model in mind, clinicians may need to think about what type of intervention an individual requires when first seen. For example, in pain management, it is often the case that the patients are required to actively engage in the treatment process. However, if the patient is not at the action stage, then immediate treatment success would not be expected. Indeed, treatment outcome research supports this model by demonstrating different success rates for a number of treatments and conditions depending on what stage of change the person is at (e.g., M. E. Jensen, Nielson, Romano, Hill, & Turner, 2000). Thus, the same treatment should not be blindly administered to everyone who is seeking some form of behavior change. Rather, as emphasized repeatedly throughout this book, treatment needs to be individually tailored to each patient's readiness of change stage. For example, patients in the precontemplation or contemplation stages should initially be provided with therapeutic strategies that will facilitate their movement into either the preparation stage or the action stage. Those in the preparation stage or the action stage should be provided more specific advice and recommendations, as well as information about how to make the behavior changes (e.g., learning coping methods to deal with pain).

Finally, it should also be pointed out that an important component of the stages-of-change model is the recognition that temporary relapse may be part of the change process. Indeed, for many patients, relapse may be predicted. These relapses can often be predicted and be prepared for so that, when they occur, the patient is ready to handle the situation. Relapse-prevention models are now routinely used in behavior change programs, such as pain management, to decrease the impact of any potential relapse and make subsequent relapse less likely to occur. Marlatt and Gordon (1985) originally proposed such relapse-prevention models, which are now viewed as important to build into any pain management program.

MOTIVATIONAL INTERVIEWING

Motivational interviewing (MI), originally developed by Miller and Rollnick (1991) for working with alcohol-dependent patients, has been applied to a variety of health behaviors, including pain. M. E. Jensen (2002) provided an excellent review of how to enhance motivation to change in the pain treatment environment. Based on Miller and Rollnick's original work, which emphasizes that patient motivation is an important component of behavior change, MI was developed as an approach to clinician–patient interaction that focuses on enhancing patients' motivation to change. MI strategies were developed to address motivational problems in patients. According to Jensen, there are a number of important issues to keep in mind when dealing with pain patients:

- An ongoing assessment of each patient's readiness-to-change stage is needed so that appropriate therapeutic strategies can be chosen specifically for that patient to enhance his or her movement through a particular change stage.
- The clinician needs to help motivate the patient to try something different from what the patient is currently doing or has tried in the past. These efforts should then be monitored in regard to how they affect the functioning of the particular patient. In this way, the clinician may help assist the patient to determine which behavior seems to be most adaptive for him or her.
- Although a basic assumption of MI is that a clinician's behavior plays a major role in the development and maintenance of patient motivation, one must keep in mind that the ultimate responsibility for change lies within the patient—that is, the clinician's major task is to enhance motivation; the patient's major task is to take action. Thus, clinicians should avoid doing anything "for" patients and place responsibility for action on the patient.

M. E. Jensen (2002) went on to summarize the five basic principles of MI originally proposed by Miller and Rollnick (1991):

1. By using the *expression of accurate empathy*, the clinician makes an effort to communicate respect for the patient and acceptance of the patient without any blame, criticism, or judgment. This includes active support for the patient's right to self-determination and direction, the ability to understand a patient's perspective, and a willingness to reflect that understanding back to the patient.

2. *Developing discrepancy* involves helping the patient develop an appropriate sense of discrepancy between his or her current behavior and important goals in his or her life. Confrontational approaches should be avoided, because they usually result in defensive patient responses. Instead, the clinician should encourage the patient to talk about the problem, listen specifically for discrepancies between patient goals and problem behaviors, and then reflect back discrepancies that are verbalized. The patient should then be encouraged to elaborate these discrepancies so that he or she becomes increasingly aware of them.

3. *Avoiding argumentation* refers to the fact that the clinician should avoid getting involved in arguing for a specific behavior change that may result in the patient arguing *against* an adaptive change. Such argumentation will often provide the patient with the opportunity to list the myriad reasons to avoid change and may therefore inhibit, rather than promote, change. If a clinician realizes that a patient is beginning to argue against some adaptive behavior change recommendation, this should be a signal for the clinician to change strategies.

4. *Rolling with resistance* refers to the fact that, by avoiding argumentation and switching strategies, the clinician needs to definitely reframe or restart the patient's comments in such a manner as to demonstrate the clinician's understanding of the patient's ambivalence about change. Often, when a clinician reflects back the patient's resistance statements, the patient may respond by taking on the other side of the argument, resulting in positive arguments for actual behavior change initially suggested.

5. *Supporting self-efficacy* involves making statements and asking questions that will stimulate the patient's hope that changes are possible. Such self-efficacy was originally defined by Bandura (1977) as the belief in one's ability to perform a specific behavior. Such positive beliefs are very therapeutic for patients.

PATIENT MOTIVATION STRATEGIES

M. E. Jensen (2002) also reviewed specific intervention strategies for pain management purposes that are consistent with the five principles of MI reviewed above. He also incorporated *motivational enhancement therapy* (MET), a three-phase intervention developed by Miller, Zweben,

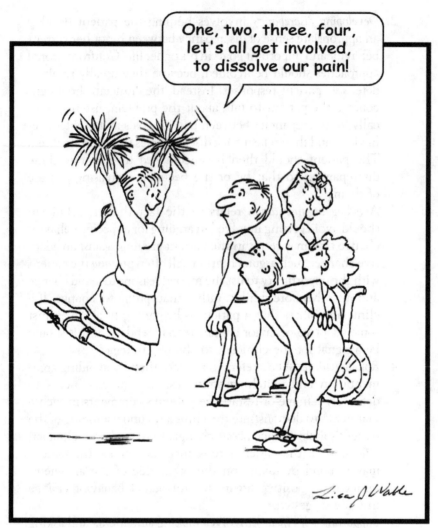

Many methods have been tried to motivate pain patients to engage in the treatment process.

DiClemente, and Rychtarik (1992). *Phase I strategies* are conceived as being best used with precontemplators and contemplators and are designed to motivate patients to consider change. *Phase II strategies* are perceived as best used with contemplators who appear to be very close to making a commitment for change; these strategies should be used to tip the balance from mere ambivalence about change to actual preparation for change. Finally, *Phase III strategies* are perceived as being used in follow-up sessions, after patients have made a strong commitment to change and have had the opportunity to take some actual action to produce this change.

MOTIVATIONAL ENHANCEMENT THERAPY STRATEGIES FOR PAIN MANAGEMENT

Phase I of MET includes the following strategies, which focus on enhancing motivation for change:

- *Eliciting self-motivational statements* from patients that acknowledge the extent and nature of the pain problem, concerns about how they are currently managing the problem, the intention of changing to more adaptive pain management methods, and optimism that such change is possible.
- *Listening with empathy,* which is important for providing a positive environment in which the clinician reflects accurately what the patient has communicated (thus acting to minimize patient resistance).
- *Questioning,* in which two techniques can be used: (a) direct questions used to elicit initial patient responses that, in turn, can be responded to with empathic listening, and (b) direct questioning to ask a series of planned questions as a method of comprehensively obtaining a great deal of specific information in a short period of time (i.e., use of a structured interview protocol).
- *Presenting personal feedback,* which involves bringing into better focus any discrepancies between what the patient is now doing to manage the pain and what the patient's personal goals and core values are (e.g., desired levels of physical functioning, social role functioning, medication use, etc.).
- *Affirming the patient* at every opportunity in the form of direct compliments and praise for any positive changes made in pain management. This further accentuates a positive environment for change by increasing rapport, the patient's self-esteem, and the patient's responsibility for change, as well as reinforcing patients' self-motivational statements.
- *Handling resistance,* which is important because patients often are reluctant to attempt any new changes for fear of an increase in pain, as well as having misinformation about what may or may not work. Clinicians will need to avoid reactions that tend to evoke resistance, such as arguing, criticizing, warning patients of possible negative consequences, confrontation, and so on.
- *Reframing* involves providing patients with feedback that presents the patient's maladaptive behavior in a generally positive light and at the same time still allows for the possibility of

more positive behavioral change. In this manner, the patient will not feel the need to have to defend his or her current pattern of behaviors, thus freeing up more energy for changing those responses.

- *Summarizing* near the end of every treatment session is important to allow patients to hear their own self-motivational statements again. The clinician should emphasize as much as possible the positive self-motivational statements made by the patient during the session.

Phase II of MET includes the following strategies, which are intended to strengthen commitment for behavior change:

- *Developing a plan for change* to which the patient can fully commit him- or herself. The clinician should attempt to elicit specific ideas and strategies for such change.
- *Communicating free choice,* which involves reminding the patient that he or she has free choice in all aspects of the behavior change plan. In this way, the clinician can facilitate the patient's attribution of control.
- *Reviewing consequences of change versus no change* will often strengthen the patient's commitment to change. The patient at this point should realize that not making any changes amounts to a life controlled by pain, as before, which the patient will regard as unsatisfactory.
- *Providing information and advice* often begins when patients start to ask for specific information and advice concerning how to proceed (e.g., Will I be pain free after completing the program? Will I have to continue exercising after I have completed the program? What should I do if my pain starts to get overwhelming after I leave the program?).
- *Rolling with resistance* is important in this phase, as it was in Phase I. One should always anticipate that patients will often have ambivalence about change during every stage of treatment.
- *Using a change plan worksheet* can provide structure for organizing the most important aspects of the patient's goals and rationale for making changes. This can serve as a reminder to patients as well as a summary after sessions concerning what goals have been met.
- *Recapitulation* involves the strategy of allowing patients to hear once again their reasons for making changes and their plans for such changes. A change plan worksheet may be used as a guide in this recapitulation process.

- *Asking for commitment*, as the phrase suggests, requests patients to commit themselves to the plan of change that they have outlined. Patients, however, should not feel pressured into making a decision of change before they are ready.

Phase III of MET consists of follow-through strategies, such as the following:

- Reviewing the overall progress made during treatment.
- If perceived as necessary, efforts to renew the patient's motivation to maintain change should be made.
- Again, if perceived as necessary, efforts to renew the patient's commitment to change should be made.

CAVEATS ABOUT MOTIVATIONAL ENHANCEMENT THERAPY

Although MI and MET were originally developed to assist problem drinkers to change their maladaptive drinking behavior, they have also been adapted for treatment of other health-related problem behaviors, such as pain. Indeed, they seem to be well suited for the treatment of pain problems because of the multiple motivational challenges that pain patients often experience in attempting to develop and maintain adaptive coping responses to their pain and disability. It is important to deal with motivational problems in all patients in order to initially enhance the effectiveness of the treatment and to address the possibility of relapse after treatment completion. As M. E. Jensen (2002) noted, these approaches are quite consistent with the biopsychosocial interdisciplinary approach to pain management, which encourages the development of adaptive behaviors such as pain coping skills, physical reconditioning and reactivation, appropriate pacing of activities, and proper use of pain medication. Recently, there have been a number of empirical investigations of such a *transtheoretical model of change* with chronic-pain patients, supporting the clinical utility of this model in persons with pain (e.g., M. E. Jensen et al., 2000; Keefe et al., 2000; Keller, Herda, Ridder, & Baseler, 2001).

MI should not be viewed as replacing educational or cognitive–behavioral interventions; rather, it is best seen as an approach that precedes these other pain management interventions and helps the patient become ready to benefit from them before they are implemented. For example, it is better for patients with chronic pain to come to the conclusion themselves that their inactivity is a major barrier to improvement they want to change than it is for the health care provider to be pushing a plan on patients who do not believe they have the time or ability to exercise. Examples of self-motivational statements to use with chronic-pain patients are presented in Appendix 7.2A.

A FINAL ADDITIONAL CLINICAL SUGGESTION

There are a number of additional ways to increase motivation and get patients fully engaged in treatment. One method that is often overlooked is to have other, "star" patients serve as your advocate. Frequently, especially in the case of chronic-pain patients, there may be a basic mistrust of health care professionals because of past disappointments in having their pain completely relieved. They are now "gun shy" and wary of new promises of improvement. However, they will be more open to hearing information and guidelines from another patient who has successfully completed the treatment program. These former patients can offer a more realistic expectation of outcomes and what the pain patient needs to overcome obstacles to cope with pain. Having such star patients come back to visit new patients can be quite inspirational and motivating. This is quite different from patients attending outside advocacy support groups, where there is often the theme propagated that a "magic cure" may be out there if the group keeps together. Such groups usually hold on to a curative philosophy of eliminating pain rather than the more appropriate illness model of managing pain. Patients usually are more receptive to information received from other patients than from physicians. It is important that this information be correct. Receiving it from patients who have successfully completed a pain management program is the only way of ensuring that the information is correct.

Providing appropriate inspirational reading material is also another good method to enhance patient motivation to "stay the course" and to develop a positive mind-set toward their currently stressful situation. Appendix 7.3 includes examples of such material.

CONCLUSIONS: A MODEL OF MOTIVATION FOR PAIN SELF-MANAGEMENT

From the preceding discussion, it is apparent that health care professionals are beginning to develop a better handle on motivation enhancement techniques and their importance in pain management. M. P. Jensen et al. (2003) also highlighted the fact that, even though no one particular technique has a clear advantage over another, there appears to be a substantial amount of overlap that exists and that may serve as the foundation for a more general model of motivation for the self-management of pain. They

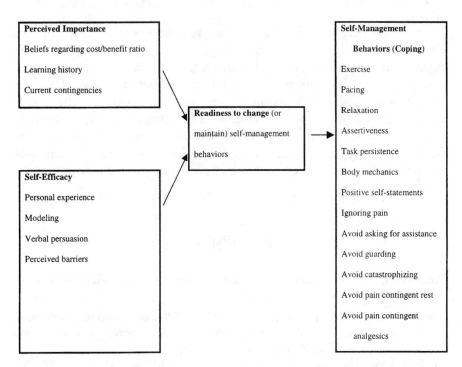

Figure 7.1. A preliminary motivational model of pain self-management. From "Toward the Development of a Motivational Model of Pain Self-Management," by M. P. Jensen, W. R. Nielson, and R. D. Kerns, 2003, *Journal of Pain, 4,* p. 484. Copyright 2003 by Guilford Press. Reprinted with permission.

provided a preliminary version of such a model, which is presented in Figure 7.1. As the reader will note, many of these concepts and techniques have been presented in this chapter and in other chapters throughout this book. Of course, additional clinical research is required to further fine tune this model and to ascertain what components are most powerful in producing the greatest degree of motivation in pain patients.

SUMMARY

The reader should keep in mind that, despite the availability of potentially effective pain management techniques, there often remain many patients who do not improve or who actually relapse. Often, this failure can be traced to low patient motivation for treatment and its compliance requirements. The stages-of-change model, reviewed in this chapter, has been shown to be a very useful conceptualization of a patient's readiness to make the necessary changes in a pain management program. If a patient is not in the action stage, then he or she may not be ready or motivated to make the necessary changes. MI has been developed to help enhance the motivation of patients to make changes in a treatment environment. Such interviewing was developed as an approach to clinician–patient interaction that focuses on enhancing patients' motivation to change. The basic principles of MI were reviewed in this chapter, and examples of the process were given. MI can be used as a motivational technique for all components of pain management, including pharmacotherapy, which I discuss in the next chapter. Finally, a more general model of motivation for pain self-management was presented that shows great promise for maximizing the motivational process.

REFERENCES

Bandura, A. (1977). Self-efficacy: Toward a unifying theory of behavioral change. *Psychological Review, 84,* 191–215.

DiClemente, C. C., & Prochaska, J. O. (1982). Self-change and therapy change of smoking behavior: A comparison of processes of change in cessation and maintenance. *Addictive Behaviors, 7,* 133–142.

Gatchel, R. J. (1991). Psychosocial assessment and disability management in the rehabilitation of painful spinal disorders. In T. Mayer, V. Mooney, & R. Gatchel (Eds.), *Contemporary conservative care for painful spinal disorders* (pp. 441–454). Philadelphia: Lea & Febiger.

Jensen, M. E. (2002). Enhancing motivation to change in pain treatment. In D. C. Turk & R. J. Gatchel (Eds.), *Psychological approaches to pain management: A practitioner's handbook* (pp. 71–93). New York: Guilford Publications.

Jensen, M. E., Nielson, W. R., Romano, J. M., Hill, M. L., & Turner, J. A. (2000). Further evaluation of the Pain Stages of Change Questionnaire: Is the transtheoretical model of change useful for patients with chronic pain? *Pain, 86,* 255–264.

Jensen, M. P., Nielson, W. R., & Kerns, R. D. (2003). Toward the development of a motivational model of pain self-management. *Journal of Pain, 4,* 477–492.

Keefe, F. J., Lefebvre, J. C., Kerns, R. D., Rosenberg, R., Beaupre, P., Prochaska, J., et al. (2000). Understanding the adoption of arthritis self-management: Stages of change profiles among arthritis patients. *Pain, 87,* 303–313.

Keller, S., Herda, C., Ridder, K., & Baseler, H. (2001). Readiness to adopt adequate postural habits: An application of the trans-theoretical model in the context of back pain prevention. *Pain Education and Counseling, 42,* 175–184.

Marlatt, G. A., & Gordon, J. R. (Eds.). (1985). *Relapse prevention: Maintenance strategies in the treatment of addictive behaviors.* New York: Guilford Press.

Miller, W. R., & Rollnick, S. (1991). *Motivational interviewing: Preparing people to change addictive behavior.* New York: Guilford Press.

Miller, W. R., Zweben, A., DiClemente, C. C., & Rychtarik, R. G. (1992). *A clinical research guide for therapists treating individuals with alcohol abuse and dependence*. Washington, DC: U.S. Government Printing Office.

Parham, A. C. (1983). *Basic psychology for the work life*. Cincinnati, OH: South-Western.

Parsons, T. (1964). *Social structure and personality*. London: Collier-MacMillan.

Pilowsky, I. (1978a). A general classification of abnormal illness behavior. *British Journal of Medical Psychiatry, 51,* 131–137.

Pilowsky, I. (1978b). Psychodynamic aspects of the pain experience. In R. A. Steinbach (Ed.), *The psychology of pain* (pp. 88–103). New York: Raven Press.

Prochaska, J. O., DiClemente, C. C., & Norcross, J. C. (1992). In search of how people change: Applications to addictive behaviors. *American Psychologist, 47,* 1102–1114.

APPENDIX 7.1

Recommended Readings

Jensen, M. E. (2002). Enhancing motivation to change in pain treatment. In D. C. Turk & R. J. Gatchel (Eds.), *Psychological approaches to pain management: A practitioner's handbook* (2nd ed., pp. 71–93). New York: Guilford Press.

Jensen, M. P., Nielson, W. R., & Kerns, R. D. (2003). Toward the development of a motivational model of pain self-management. *Journal of Pain, 4,* 477–492.

Miller, W. R., & Rollnick, S. (1991). *Motivational interviewing: Preparing people to change addictive behavior.* New York: Guilford Press.

APPENDIX 7.2A

Examples of Self-Motivational Statements With Chronic-Pain Patients

Problem Recognition

- "Perhaps I'm neglecting my overall problem with pain more than I realized."
- "I can see that, over the years, my problem with pain is going to lead to more serious problems."
- "Maybe I have not been doing the right things."

Expressions of Concern

- "I'm really worried about this."
- "How could I let myself go like this?"
- "I don't know how people do this."

Intention to Change

- "How do people deal with their pain every day? I've got to figure this out."
- "I want to control my pain better. What can I do?"
- "I don't know how I'm going to do it, but I've got to control my pain."

Optimism About Change

- "I know I can help to control my pain if I just put my mind to it."
- "Other people control their pain; I know I can, too."
- "I think I can start exercising more to help control my pain; it'll be worth it in the long run."

APPENDIX 7.2B

Strategies for Handling Resistance

Simple Reflection

Definition: Acknowledgment of the patient's disagreement, emotion, or perception.

Example:
Patient: All you doctors are trying to tell me how to live my life. I'm sick of it.
Provider: You're tired of people telling you what you should do and not do.

Amplified Reflection

Definition: Reflecting back what the patient said in an amplified or exaggerated form.

Example:
Patient: I can't do all these things to keep my pain controlled. It's just too hard.
Provider: So you don't feel you can make changes in any area of your life right now.

Double-Sided Reflection

Definition: Acknowledging what the patient said and adding to it the other side of the ambivalence.

Example:
Patient: Almost every one of my friends who have some pain don't practice stress management. I don't see what the big deal is. They're doing fine.
Provider: It sounds like, on the one hand, you see the importance of sticking to the recommendations to try to practice stress management more to help your pain. On the other hand, however, you see others with pain not practicing it and not having any problems. That's hard to figure out.

Shifting Focus

Definition: Shifting the patient's attention away from what seems to be a stumbling block standing in the way of progress.

Example:
Patient: I know you want me to practice stress management on a regular basis to help my pain, but I can't do it. I'm just not going to do it!
Provider: OK, let's not get ahead of ourselves. The most important thing is that we keep you relaxed and manage your pain, doing the things you

want to do. How we best do that is something we need to figure out as we go along. So let's not get stuck in the details yet. What I think we should do first is give you some information about what different stress management programs there are and look for some of the things you might feel you can do on a regular basis. OK?

Agreement With a Twist

Definition: Offering initial agreement, but with a slight twist or change of direction.

Example:
Patient: You tell me I may be able to help decrease my pain somewhat if I practice stress management, but you don't understand how hard that is. No one I know practices it.
Provider: You've got a good point there. Like we've discussed, stress management can make a difference, but it's certainly not as simple as that. I agree with you on that.

Emphasizing Personal Choice

Definition: Reassuring patients that, in the end, they will determine what happens.

Example:
Patient: All of these changes you are telling me I need to make—it's not like it is certain to reduce my pain. I really don't know about all of this.
Provider: We've discussed some of the pros and cons of making some lifestyle changes. I can't decide for you what you are going to do, however. It's really up to you to decide.

Reframing

Definition: Acknowledging the validity of the patient's observations but offering a new interpretation for them.

Example:
Patient: My wife is always annoyed at me when I complain about my pain and stress level. She never gives me a break! I get so angry I want to go to the emergency room just to get back at her.
Provider: It sounds like she really cares about you and wants you to be healthy. I guess she expresses it in a way that you're angry about. Maybe we can help her find a more helpful way of expressing her concern about you.

APPENDIX 7.3A

Be Aware of the Snowball Effect of Your Thinking

A powerful technique for becoming more peaceful is to be aware of how quickly your negative and insecure thinking can spiral out of control. Have you ever noticed how uptight you feel when you're caught up in your thinking? And, to top it off, the more absorbed you get in the details of whatever is upsetting you, the worse you feel. One thought leads to another, and yet another, until at some point, you become incredibly agitated.

For example, you might wake up in the middle of the night and remember a phone call that needs to be made the following day. Then, rather than feeling relieved that you remembered such an important call, you start thinking about everything else you have to do tomorrow. You start rehearsing a probable conversation with your boss, getting yourself even more upset. Pretty soon you think to yourself, "I can't believe how busy I am. I must make fifty phone calls a day. Whose life is this anyway?" and on and on it goes until you're feeling sorry for yourself. For many people, there's no limit to how long this type of "thought attack" can go on. In fact, I've been told by clients that many of their days and nights are spent in this type of mental rehearsal. Needless to say, it's impossible to feel peaceful with your head full of concerns and annoyances.

The solution is to notice what's happening in your head before your thoughts have a chance to build any momentum. The sooner you catch yourself in the act of building your mental snowball, the easier it is to stop. In our example here, you might notice your snowball thinking right when you start running through the list of what you have to do the next day. Then, instead of obsessing on your upcoming day, you say to yourself, "Whew, there I go again," and consciously nip it in the bud. You stop your train of thought before it has a chance to get going. You can then focus, not on how overwhelmed you are, but on how grateful you are for remembering the phone call that needed to be made. If it's the middle of the night, write it down on a piece of paper and go back to sleep. You might even consider keeping a pen and paper by the bed for such moments.

You may indeed be a very busy person, but remember that filling your head with thoughts of how overwhelmed you are only exacerbates the problem by making you feel even more stressed than you already do. Try this simple little exercise next time you begin to obsess on your schedule. You'll be amazed at how effective it can be.

Note. Handout for patients suffering from stress. From *Don't Sweat the Small Stuff . . . And It's All Small Stuff* (pp. 13–15), by R. Carlson, 1997, New York: Hyperion. Copyright 1997 by Hyperion Press. Reprinted with permission.

APPENDIX 7.3B

Think of Your Problems as Potential Teachers

Most people would agree that one of the greatest sources of stress in our lives is our problems. To a certain degree this is true. A more accurate assessment, however, is that the amount of stress we feel has more to do with how we relate to our problems than it does with the problems themselves. In other words, how much of a problem do we make our problems? Do we see them as emergencies, or as potential teachers?

Problems come in many shapes, sizes, and degrees of seriousness, but all have one thing in common: They present us with something that we wish were different. The more we struggle with our problems and the more we want them to go away, the worse they seem and the more stress they cause us.

Ironically, and luckily, the opposite is also true. When we accept our problems as an inevitable part of life, when we look at them as potential teachers, it's as if a weight has been lifted off our shoulders.

Think of a problem that you have struggled with for quite some time. How have you dealt with this problem up until now? If you're like most, you've probably struggled with it, mentally rehearsed it, analyzed it again and again, but have come up short. Where has all this struggle led you? Probably to even more confusion and stress.

Now think of the problem in a new way. Rather than push away the problem and resist it, try to embrace it. Mentally, hold the problem near to your heart. Ask yourself what valuable lesson(s) this problem might be able to teach you. Could it be teaching you to be more careful or patient? Does it have anything to do with greed, envy, carelessness, or forgiveness? Or something equally powerful? Whatever problems you are dealing with, chances are they could be thought of in a softer way that includes a genuine desire to learn from them. When you hold your problems in this light, they soften like a clenched fist that is opening. Give this strategy a try, and I think you'll agree that most problems aren't the emergencies we think they are. And usually, once we learn what we need to learn, they begin to go away.

Note. Handout for patients suffering from stress. From *Don't Sweat the Small Stuff . . . And It's All Small Stuff* (pp. 13–15), by R. Carlson, 1997, New York: Hyperion. Copyright 1997 by Hyperion Press. Reprinted with permission.

APPENDIX 7.3C

Become More Patient

The quality of patience goes a long way toward your goal of creating a more peaceful and loving self. The more patient you are, the more accepting you will be of what is, rather than insisting that life be exactly as you would like it to be. Without patience, life is extremely frustrating. You are easily annoyed, bothered, and irritated. Patience adds a dimension of ease and acceptance to your life. It's essential for inner peace.

Becoming more patient involves opening your heart to the present moment, even if you don't like it. If you are stuck in a traffic jam, late for an appointment, opening to the moment would mean catching yourself building a mental snowball before your thinking got out of hand and gently reminding yourself to relax. It might also be a good time to breathe as well as an opportunity to remind yourself that, in the bigger scheme of things, being late is "small stuff."

Patience also involves seeing the innocence in others. My wife, Kris, and I have two young children ages four and seven. On many occasions while writing this book, our four-year-old daughter has walked into my office and interrupted my work, which can be disruptive to a writer. What I have learned to do (most of the time) is to see the innocence in her behavior rather than to focus on the potential implications of her interruption ("I won't get my work done, I'll lose my train of thought, this was my only opportunity to write today," and so forth). I remind myself *why* she is coming to see me—because she loves me, not because she is conspiring to ruin my work. When I remember to see the innocence, I immediately bring forth a feeling of patience, and my attention is brought back to the moment. Any irritation that may have been building is eliminated and I'm reminded, once again, of how fortunate I am to have such beautiful children. I have found that, if you look deeply enough, you can almost always see the innocence in other people as well as in potentially frustrating situations. When you do, you will become a more patient and peaceful person and, in some strange way, you begin to enjoy many of the moments that used to frustrate you.

Note. Handout for patients suffering from stress. From *Don't Sweat the Small Stuff . . . And It's All Small Stuff* (pp. 13–15), by R. Carlson, 1997, New York: Hyperion. Copyright 1997 by Hyperion Press. Reprinted with permission.

APPENDIX 7.3D

Make Peace With Imperfection

I've yet to meet an absolute perfectionist whose life was filled with inner peace. The need for perfection and the desire for inner tranquility conflict with each other. Whenever we are attached to having something a certain way, better than it already is, we are, almost by definition, engaged in a losing battle. Rather than being content and grateful for what we have, we are focused on what's wrong with something and our need to fix it. When we are zeroed in on what's wrong, it implies that we are dissatisfied, discontent.

Whether it's related to ourselves—a disorganized closet, a scratch on the car, an imperfect accomplishment, a few pounds we would like to lose—or of someone else's "imperfections"—the way someone looks, behaves, or lives their life—the very act of focusing on imperfection pulls us away from our goal of being kind and gentle. This strategy has nothing to do with ceasing to do your very best but with being overly attached and focused on what's wrong with life. It's about realizing that while there's always a better way to do something, this doesn't mean that you can't enjoy and appreciate the way things already are.

The solution here is to catch yourself when you fall into your habit of insisting that things should be other than they are. Gently remind yourself that life is okay the way it is, right now. In the absence of your judgment, everything would be fine. As you begin to eliminate your need for perfection in all areas of your life, you'll begin to discover the perfection in life itself.

Note. Handout for patients suffering from stress. From *Don't Sweat the Small Stuff . . . And It's All Small Stuff* (pp. 13–15), by R. Carlson, 1997, New York: Hyperion. Copyright 1997 by Hyperion Press. Reprinted with permission.

APPENDIX 7.3E

Attitude

The longer I live, the more I realize the impact of attitude on life. Attitude, to me, is more important than facts. It is more important than the past, than education, than money, than circumstances, than failures, than successes, than what other people think or say or do. It is more important than appearance, giftedness or skill. It will make or break a company . . . a church . . . a home.

The remarkable thing is we have a choice every day regarding the attitude we will embrace for that day.

We can not change our past . . . we can not change the fact that people will act in a certain way. We can not change the inevitable. The only thing we can do is play on the one string we have, and that is our attitude. I am convinced that life is 10% what happens to me and 90% how I react to it. And so it is with you . . . we are in charge of our attitudes!

—Charles Swindall (http://www.greatest-quotations.com)

Note. Handout for patients suffering from stress.

APPENDIX 7.3F

Happiness

Sadly, many of us continually postpone our happiness indefinitely. It's not that we consciously set out to do so, but that we keep convincing ourselves, "Some day I'll be happy."

We tell ourselves we'll be happy when our bills are paid, when we get out of school, get our first job, a promotion. We convince ourselves that life will be better after we get married, have a baby, then another. Then we are frustrated that the kids aren't old enough, we'll be more content when they are. After that, we're frustrated that we have teenagers to deal with. We will certainly be happy when they are out of that stage. We tell ourselves that our life will be complete when our spouse gets his or her act together, when we get a nice car, are able to go on a nice vacation, when we retire.

The truth is, there's no better time to be happy than right now. If not now, when?

Your life will always be filled with challenges. It's best to admit this to yourself and decide to be happy anyway. Alfred D'Souza wrote, "For a long time it had seemed to me that real life was about to begin. But there was always some obstacle in the way, something to be gotten through first, some unfinished business, time still to be served, a debt to be paid. Then life would begin. At last it dawned on me that these obstacles were my life." This perspective has helped me to see that there is no way to happiness. Happiness is the way. So, treasure every moment you have! And treasure it more because you shared it with someone special, special enough to spend your time with. And remember that time waits for no one.

Yesterday is history

Tomorrow is a mystery

Today is a gift

That's why it's called the present!

So, stop waiting until you finish school, until you go back to school, until you lose ten pounds, until you gain ten pounds, until you have kids, until your kids leave the house, until you start work, until you retire, until you get married, until you get divorced, until Friday night, until Sunday morning, until you get a new car or home, until your car or home is paid off, until spring, until summer, until fall, until you are off welfare, until the first or fifteenth, until "your song" comes on, until you've had a drink, until you've sobered up, until you die, until you are born again to decide that there is no better time than right now to be happy.

Happiness is a journey . . . not a destination.

Note. Handout for patients suffering from stress. The material in this section is from "Enhancing Motivation to Change in Pain Treatment," by M. E. Jensen, in *Psychological Approaches to Pain Management: A Practitioner's Handbook* (pp. 71–93), edited by D. C. Turk and R. J. Gatchel, 2002, New York: Guilford Press. Copyright 2002 by Guilford Press. Adapted with permission.

8

PHARMACOTHERAPY

When you seek relief from headache with an aspirin, social relaxation
with alcohol, or any other drug-induced alteration of your physical or
psychological state, the drug you use must somehow get from the external
world into your body and ultimately to the specific site within the body
or brain where it can exert its effect. . . . Simple though this may sound,
transporting a drug from outside the body to its ultimate site of action
is a complex process.

—R. M. Julien (1981)

Most frequently, the first step in the treatment of pain is the use of a
host of pharmaceutical agents. In fact, data from the pharmaceutical industry
reveal that more than 312 million prescriptions for analgesic medication
were written in the year 2000 alone in the United States (Turk, in press).
In addition, pain medications are the second most prescribed drugs during
physician office and emergency room visits (Schappert, 1998). They account
for 12% of all medications that are prescribed during ambulatory visits
(National Center for Health Statistics, 1998).

With the above statistics in mind, in this chapter I review the many
classes of drugs with documented efficacy in controlling pain, as initially
outlined by Polatin and Gajraj (2002). Early or acute pain is usually treated
aggressively, with agents that act directly either on the anatomical sites of
the pain or on the central receptors. The initial focus is on reducing the
intensity of the primary nociceptive symptom. However, the longer the pain
lasts, the more complicated the treatment process may become. As the pain
process continues, other pharmacological agents may be used and act on
the transmission or augmentation of the nociceptive signal to the nervous
system and on the secondary symptoms that may develop with chronicity.
For example, the psychotropic agents, particularly the antidepressants, have
a well-documented role in the management of chronic pain. Often, *rational
polypharmacology* (i.e., the use of multiple medications) needs to be combined
with interdisciplinary treatment when managing chronic pain.

ISSUES OF TOLERANCE, DEPENDENCE, ABUSE, AND WITHDRAWAL IN PHARMACOTHERAPY

Before I review the various medication regimens that may be used in pain management, I discuss the issues of tolerance, dependence, abuse, and withdrawal, because they are concerns with regard to some pharmacological agents used to treat pain, particularly the opioids, the stimulants, and the minor tranquilizers (anxiolytics). As Polatin and Gajraj (2002) and Harden (2002) have noted, *tolerance* refers to the need to increase the dose of a drug over time to achieve the same effects; that is, it is a physiological adaptive process. Tolerance is usually not a major clinical problem with most patients, except those who may be prone to addiction. Such patients, though, can be identified by initial careful biopsychosocial assessment and conscientious clinical monitoring. *Dependence* refers to the array of symptoms that may be precipitated by the cessation of a particular drug. Such dependence may range from mild restlessness to severe manifestations, such as seizures or coma, if certain drugs are completely and suddenly stopped. *Addiction* is more of a behavioral phenomenon, referring to the aberrant use of a substance in a manner characterized by behaviors such as the preoccupation with obtaining and using the drug (i.e., obsession and compulsion about drug use), loss of control, and the resultant social and occupational problems and impairment. *Abuse* is a term used to characterize the maladaptive pattern of psychoactive substance use outside the conventional sociocultural norms or when therapeutic indications for the need of a drug are not present. In the United States, all use of illicit drugs is considered abuse, as is the use of drugs not according to a physician's prescribed orders. Legal, regulatory measures from outside the medical profession have been instituted in this country to minimize the risks of abuse, and they exercise a significant influence on the prescribing practices of physicians. Currently, abuse for any drug is evaluated according to its use for both physical and psychological dependence. Within this schema, there are five classes of drugs: Schedule I, II, III, IV, and V. *Schedule I* drugs are those with the greatest abuse potential, with no accepted medical use (such as cocaine and heroin). The potential for abuse decreases with each increasing stage, so that *Schedule V* drugs are those with the lowest potential for abuse. The various opioid prescription medications are classified as *Schedule II, III, and IV* drugs.

It should also be pointed out that, according to the American Pain Society (1992), the inconsistent use of the term *addiction* has resulted in a frequent misunderstanding among health care providers, patients, and the general public concerning the appropriate use of medications in pain management. As a result, pain may often be undertreated, and patients may be inappropriately stigmatized because of their medical use of opioids (Liaison Committee on Pain and Addiction, 2001). To address the discrepancies in the definition of opioid addiction among chronic-pain patients, three national organizations (the American Academy of Pain Medicine, the American Pain Society, and the American Society of Addiction to Medicine) developed a consensus definition of *addiction* as related to pain patients being treated with opioids:

> primary, chronic, neurobiological disease, with genetic, psychosocial and environmental factors influencing its development and manifestations. It is characterized by behaviors that include one of the following: impaired control over drug use, compulsive use, continued use despite harm, and craving. (Liaison Committee on Pain and Addiction, 2001)

As a general rule of thumb, patients who are likely to do well on controlled substances in a primary-care practice have the following characteristics:

- They are generally goal oriented and adherent to medical regimens.
- They are functional.
- They take responsibility for health outcomes and their role in multimodality treatment.
- They understand concepts in opioid use, such as tolerance, dependency, and addiction.
- There is an absence of severe chronic psychopathology.
- There is an absence of a serious personality disorder.
- They rarely overuse medications.
- There is no history of illicit drug or alcohol abuse.

Finally, besides the potentially serious physiological and behavioral syndromes just discussed, there may be other potentially negative side effects of a particular pharmacological agent (e.g., central nervous system depression, toxicity to liver or kidney functioning, etc.). A more comprehensive review of addiction and pain assessment and treatment issues was provided by Jamison (2002). Finally, Cole (2003) and Oliver and Taylor (2003) have presented excellent overviews of ground rules to follow when prescribing controlled substances.

One way of potentially avoiding problems with possible medication abuse is to address the issue at the start of any intervention. A medication agreement can help achieve this by clearly stating the responsibility of the patient not to misuse any drugs and having the patient sign a contract to that effect. In passing, it should be noted that the term *agreement* should be used rather than *contract*, because the latter implies a legal document (which it is not). One such agreement that my colleagues and I have used is presented in Appendix 8.2. In addition to the agreement, it is also useful to have a handout to give to patients to remind them of the medication refill policy of the center or clinic. This will help save valuable front-office staff time fielding questions about medication refills. Appendix 8.3 includes an example of such a handout. It should also be pointed out that there have been some recent psychometrically sound self-report instruments developed to flag patients who may have a tendency to misuse opioids (Adams et al., 2004; see Appendix 8.4)

INTEGRATION OF PHARMACOTHERAPY WITH THE OVERALL BIOPSYCHOSOCIAL TREATMENT OF PAIN

As stated earlier, acute pain is usually treated aggressively. The choice of a particular medication often proceeds from a weaker to a stronger agent, depending on the clinical response of the patient. For example, an initial trial with a nonsteroidal anti-inflammatory drug (NSAID) may be tried. If the patient shows a poor response to this medication, then one might proceed to a weak opioid, such as codeine or hydrocodone. If there is no relief from this medication, then a stronger opioid, such as morphine, oxycodone, or methadone, may be prescribed. Because of legal concerns of psychological dependence and potential abuse, many physicians are hesitant to use opioids except in the case of patients with very poor prognoses, such as cancer pain. Indeed, even in acute-pain patients, surveys have shown that physicians usually underprescribe the opioids (Cooper, Czechowicz, Peterson, & Molinan, 1992), with doses that are suboptimal, too infrequent, or for inadequate periods of time. Thus, many acute-pain patients who see not pain specialists, but rather primary-care physicians, may not be adequately treated at the early stages of their pain.

If the acute pain episode is not treated effectively, there is always the great potential for chronic pain to develop. At this point, treatment becomes much more complex. Pharmacotherapy is still an important treatment approach in managing pain, but it will best be used in a multidisciplinary context, in conjunction with other biopsychosocial interventions focused on decreasing suffering and increasing functioning (as discussed in earlier chapters). One cannot assume that medication alone will resolve the complex biopsychosocial factors associated with a chronic-pain patient. It is at this stage that a pain specialist must be knowledgeable about the various choices of medication available to control pain: the dosage ranges, and the potential side effects, as well as the efficacy of specific drugs for various pain syndromes. For example, when pain becomes chronic, its experience may differ depending on the site and nature of the pathophysiology. Cluster headaches are descriptively different from muscle tension or migraine headaches. This basic nociceptive difference would be expected to be associated with variations and efficacy of different drugs. For example, the opioids, although they are the most universally effective pain medications, are less effective with neuropathic syndromes and bone pain (Twycross, 1994). There is a tendency for neuropathic pain to be relatively opioid resistant, but it responds much better to antidepressant and anticonvulsant medications. Bone pain, in turn, responds better to NSAIDs. These various drugs are reviewed in more detail later in this chapter.

It should also be pointed out that there are often secondary symptoms of emotional distress seen in patients who have chronic pain that will worsen the prognosis for improvement unless they are adequately treated. Indeed, studies have consistently documented high rates of major depression, anxiety disorders, and substance abuse problems in chronic-pain patients (e.g., Dersh, Polatin, & Gatchel, 2002). Psychopharmacological agents will, therefore, often be required to treat secondary symptoms of emotional distress in these patients. Such polypharmacology will require that all medications be carefully prescribed and monitored so as not to counter the effects of pain medications that are concurrently prescribed.

PHARMACOLOGICAL AGENTS USED TO TREAT PAIN

Polatin and Gajraj (2002) and Cole (2002) have provided excellent reviews of the major pharmacological agents that can be used to treat pain. These agents are discussed below. It should also be noted that there are potentially different routes of administration of various medications, including the following (J. Painter, personal communication, 2003):

- Oral
- Sublingual/buccal
- Intravenous dose = subcutaneous dose
- Transdermal (patch), which takes 17 to 24 hours to achieve an appropriate plasma level
- Rectal
- Intrathecal/epidural
- Nebulized

Moreover, there are various factors to consider regarding the best route of administration:

- Venous access
- Epidural/intrathecal
- Oral route, which requires gastrointestinal functioning
- Intravenous/subcutaneous/rectal administration avoids primary pass of the liver

TABLE 8.1
Commonly Used Opioids and Their Centrally Acting Analgesic Dosages

Drug name	Oral dosage (mg)
Morphine	30
Codeine	200
Hydrocodone (Lortab)	5–10
Hydromorphone (Dilaudid)	2–4
Levo-Dromoran	2
Methadone	20
Oxycodone	30
Meperidine	300
Pentazocine	120
Tramadol (Ultram)	50–100
OxyContin	10–40
Morphine Sustained Release Contin	15–60
Duragesic patch (Fentanyl)	25–100 micrograms

Common side effects of opioids

Type of effect	Symptom(s)
Central nervous system	Drowsiness, mood changes, suppressed cough, respiratory depression, miosis or "mental clouding"
Cardiovascular	Orthostatic hypotension
Gastrointestinal	Abdominal pain, constipation, nausea and vomiting
Other	Urinary retention; sweating, flushing, and itching; tolerance; addiction; withdrawal

Note. From "Integration of Pharmacotherapy With Psychological Treatment of Chronic Pain," by P. B. Polatin and N. M. Gajraj, in *Psychological Approaches to Pain Management: A Practitioner's Handbook* (2nd ed., pp. 276–298), edited by D. C. Turk and R. J. Gatchel, 2002, New York: Guilford Press. Copyright 2002 by Guilford Press. Adapted with permission.

- Sublingual/buccal avoids primary pass of the liver
- Transdermal indications for use
- Does the patient fear needle injections?

Opioids

As I review in the next chapter, after all other treatments have failed to help a patient to experience some degree of pain relief and to regain function, *palliative care* is considered (with opioids being a primary medication involved in such care). However, opioids can also be used in earlier stages of pain management. Because they are widely used, a more detailed discussion of them is provided here. A list of commonly used opioids and centrally acting analgesic dosages, as well as a summary of some of the common side effects of opioids in general, is presented in Table 8.1. In passing, one should also be aware of the conversion of oral and intravenous (IV) narcotics:

- Morphine oral dose = 3 times the IV dose
- Morphine IV dose = 1/3 oral dose
- Morphine and oxycodone = 1:1 conversion
- Morphine 10 mg = Demerol 75 mg
- Dilaudid dose = 1/6 of morphine dose

Polatin and Gajraj (2002) indicated that the opioids are the most beneficial medications for the relief of pain because of their primary agonistic effects on opioidal receptors in the brain and the spinal cord. As indicated earlier, though, surveys have shown that physicians usually underprescribe opioids, even in acute-pain patients, because of legal concerns about possible addiction and abuse. However, investigations of even long-term treatment with opioids for chronic pain have indicated a very low risk of addiction in patients who have an absence of factors such as past history of substance abuse or severe personality disorders (e.g., Portenoy & Foley, 1986). Another common concern of physicians is the potential for respiratory depression or arrest caused by opioids. However, clinical research has indicated that pain actually physiologically antagonizes the central depressive effects of opioids (Twycross, 1994); this side effect, though, can readily be seen in an addict or control participant who does not have clinical pain. Most pain management specialists realize that, even at high doses of potent narcotics used with chronic-pain patients, careful medical monitoring of the patients will decrease any significant risk of respiratory depression.

Polatin and Gajraj (2002) presented guidelines that were developed for the administration of opioid maintenance therapy to patients with chronic, noncancer pain. These include the following:

- Administration of prior trials of some nonopioid analgesia to determine pain relief effectiveness.
- Exclusion of patients who have a high risk for addiction (which, again, can be determined by a comprehensive biopsychosocial evaluation).
- Having a single physician take the primary responsibility for the opioid medication.
- Documentation that the pain syndrome being treated is responsive to opioids by a clinical trial that is carefully documented.
- Specific goals for functional improvement, as well as pain relief, should be clearly stipulated and agreed on by the patient to justify the medication regimen.

- On a regular basis, there should be careful monitoring and documentation of the degree of analgesia, any side effects, functional status, and evidence of any aberrant drug-related behavior.
- In terms of the administration of opioid medications, it has been suggested that, for maximum patient comfort, the dosing intervals should not be on an as-needed basis because, by the time pain re-emerges, the patient would have had an interval of discomfort prior to the therapeutic onset of the next dose. Instead, it is recommended that patients should be dosed on a time-contingent basis. This time-contingent basis is determined by the half-life of the particular medication; this may range, for example, from 2 hours for Demerol to 8 hours for Methadone. Drugs with shorter half-lives, such as Demerol and Pentazocine, will require much more frequent dosing and are less desirable for the treatment of chronic pain.
- The choice of a particular medication should always proceed from a weaker agent to a stronger one, depending on the patient's clinical response. In opioid-responsive pain, a patient will usually plateau at a particular dose level, beyond which further increase will not be required to control his or her pain. Of course, side effects of opioids, as presented in Table 8.1, must be monitored. For example, constipation is quite common, but it can be controlled easily by laxatives. Geriatric patients are usually at a higher risk for oversedation, urinary retention, and hypotension; however, with careful monitoring of dosage and side effects, they may still be effectively managed for chronic-pain complaints.

Shanti, Tan, and Shenaq (2001) highlighted the fact that, for patients experiencing some unwanted side effects from opioids, then switching the delivery and type of the pharmaceutical administered can often lead to greater pain relief.

Non-Narcotic Analgesics

Again, as Polatin and Gajraj (2002) presented, the major effects of a non-narcotic analgesic are at the tissue site of the pain, even though there may be certain centrally mediated effects as well. Treatment efficacy is mostly proven in those pain syndromes associated with inflammatory processes, such as rheumatoid arthritis and osteoarthritis. They may also be beneficial for short-term management of musculoskeletal pain and headaches and are also an ideal initial choice for the control of mild to moderate acute pain. In chronic-pain syndromes of central peripheral origin, however, there is much

TABLE 8.2
Commonly Used Nonsteroidal Anti-Inflammatory Drug Dosage Levels

Drug name	Dosage level (mg)
Fenoprofen (Nalfon)	200–600
Flurbibrofen (Ansaid)	100
Ibuprofen (Motrin)	400–800
Naproxen (Naprosyn)	350–500
Oxaprozin (Daypro)	600–1200
Etodolac (Lodine)	300–600
Indomethacin (Indocin)	25–75
Piroxicam (Feldene)	10–20
Celecoxib (Celebrex)	100–200
Rofecoxib (Vioxx)	12.5–50

Note. Brand names are in parentheses. From "Integration of Pharmacotherapy With Psychological Treatment of Chronic Pain," by P. B. Polatin and N. M. Gajraj, in *Psychological Approaches to Pain Management: A Practitioner's Handbook* (2nd ed., pp. 276–298), edited by D. C. Turk and R. J. Gatchel, 2002, New York: Guilford Press. Copyright 2002 by Guilford Press. Adapted with permission.

more controversy concerning their utility. Overall, this group of drugs includes medications such as aspirin, acetaminophen (e.g., Tylenol), and the NSAIDs. Some of the common NSAIDs are listed in Table 8.2. It should be noted that regular use of high doses of NSAIDs over a long period may cause injury to the stomach and intestines of some individuals, and therefore they need to be carefully monitored (although, according to the Food and Drug Administration [FDA], only 2% to 4% of patients using them a year or more suffer such complications).

Many non-narcotic analgesics can be administered once a day, thus making them much more convenient for responsive patients. Because such drugs have a ceiling effect, increasing the dosage above a certain threshold will not increase analgesia, although it may increase duration of pain relief. NSAIDs produce analgesia by blocking the actions of cyclo-oxygenase (COX) enzymes, which facilitate prostaglandin biosynthesis involved in the normal inflammatory response that causes nociceptive stimulation of different nerves, resulting in pain. Prostaglandins are a group of naturally occurring fatty acids that stimulate contraction of smooth muscle. COX activity, in turn, is associated with two different isoenzymes: (a) COX-1, which protects the stomach lining against acid-related damage, and (b) COX-2, which is involved in pathophysiologic processes such as inflammation and associated pain. Traditional NSAIDs block the action of both isoenzymes and are therefore associated with a higher incidence of epigastric side effects because of their blockade of COX-1 activity. In the late 1990s, the FDA approved the first COX-2 specific inhibitor (Celebrex), which has analgesic efficacy comparable to conventional NSAIDs but does not affect the protective epigastric activity of COX-1. The FDA subsequently approved two other COX-2 inhibitors: Vioxx and Bextra.

Again, any medication may be associated with side effects. Side effects of NSAIDs are frequent, particularly in the gastrointestinal tract (Polatin & Gajraj, 2002). There may be irritation of the stomach, lower esophagus, and colon. This irritation, in turn, may cause symptoms such as indigestion and heartburn, as well as diarrhea that may progress to the passage of blood in stool or vomitus. Moreover, with a prolonged therapeutic regimen, elevation of liver function tests may occur, although it rarely progresses to tissue damage. Other potential side effects are the following: prolonged bleeding time; easy bruising; impaired kidney function; photosensitivity; bronchospasm; worsening of asthma; and occasional central nervous system effects, such as headache, tinnitus, and some hearing loss. Thus, careful medical monitoring of these medications is essential. However, one side effect that is not seen with these medications is dependence or addiction, thereby making such drugs much more popular for the treatment of chronic pain, even though their clinical efficacy might not be as great.

In terms of the selection of the best NSAID to use, the usual method is that if one drug does not work, then the next choice should be from a different chemical group. Moreover, before the NSAIDs are rejected for ineffectiveness, trials of at least four different agents should be attempted, with 2 weeks on each drug, as well as administration on a regularly scheduled, time-contingent dosage basis (Polatin & Gajraj, 2002). In addition, while these medications are being taken, patients should be routinely questioned about any side effects and should have their bleeding time, and liver and kidney function tests, performed at regular intervals.

Antidepressants

Antidepressants are often used in the treatment of chronic-pain disorders (Hochman, Anderson, & Tennant, 2003). They are most commonly used for headache and neuropathic pain, and less so in arthritis and low back pain. There is still much debate concerning whether antidepressants produce improvement in such chronic-pain disorders by a direct antinociceptive effect or by the lessening of the secondary symptom of depression that is so commonly present in chronic-pain patients (Hochman et al., 2003). A number of clinical studies, however, have documented a direct analgesic property of these medications. In general, antidepressants can be divided into two broad categories (Exhibit 8.1). The *heterocyclics* exert their main therapeutic effect by blockading the reuptake of biogenic amines (i.e., biologically produced chemicals, such as adrenaline) in the central nervous system and the spinal cord. The two amines most closely involved in depression and chronic pain are norepinephrine and serotonin. The heterocyclics vary in their specificity for either one or both of these amines. The other major category—the *monoamine oxydase (MAO) inhibitors,* which inhibit

EXHIBIT 8.1
Two Major Categories of Antidepressants

Heterocyclics	Monoamine Oxydase Inhibitors
Amitriptyline (Elavil)	Isocarboxazid (Marplan)
Amoxapine (Asendin)	Phenelzine (Nardil)
Bupropion (Wellbutrin)	Tranylcypromine (Parnate)
Citalopram (Celexa)	
Clompramine (Anafranil)	
Desipramine (Norpramin)	
Doxepin (Sinequan)	
Fluoxetine (Prozac)	
Imipramine (Trofanil)	
Maprotiline (Ludiomil)	
Mirtazapine (Remeron)	
Nortriptyline (Pamelor)	
Paroxetine (Paxil)	
Sertraline (Zoloft)	
Trazodone (Desyrel)	
Venlafaxine (Effexor)	

Note. Brand names are in parentheses.

the impact of certain enzymes—act on a different metabolic pathway. They inhibit the enzyme MAO in the brain, thereby blocking the degradation of the biogenic amines. In clinical practice, this general category of agents is less desirable than the heterocyclics because of the potential risk of severe hypertension that can be caused by the effect of certain foods and pharmacological agents on the MAO-inhibited patient. Therefore, patients on MAO inhibitors must be on a tyramine-free diet, and they must also avoid a number of other prescriptions and over-the-counter medications. Tyramine is structurally related to epinephrine and norepinephrine and has similar actions, such as vasoconstruction. It is found in food substances such as aged cheese and red wine. These MAO inhibitors, nevertheless, have been shown to be effective in relieving migraine headache and atypical facial pain, as well as the symptoms of depression.

It should also be noted that there are often side effects of heterocyclic antidepressants that require careful clinical monitoring (Polatin & Gajraj, 2002). These side effects may include primary autonomic (e.g., dry mouth, insomnia, urinary retention, retarded ejaculation), cardiac (e.g., postural hypotension, tachycardia or elevated heart rate, arrhythmias), ocular (e.g., blurred vision, glaucoma), gastric (e.g., constipation, heartburn, nausea) and central nervous system (sedation and hangover effects, headaches, agitation, withdrawal syndrome) symptoms. Therefore, careful clinical monitoring is required. Dosage levels of all heterocyclics should be started low and tritrated upward, guided by improvement in pain or depression and by emergence of any possible side effects. For several of the older tricylics (e.g., Elavil,

Sinequan, and Tofranil), a therapeutic blood level is associated with some dry mouth or morning hangover. However, if any side effect is associated with distress or impaired functioning, a dosage modification, or an actual change of the medication, will be needed.

Of course, the evaluation for depression should occur prior to the administration of any antidepressant therapy. As Polatin and Gajraj (2002) noted, a number of characteristics of these antidepressants should be kept in mind:

- Even though all heterocyclics have antidepressant effects, some have more of a medicating effect on chronic pain, particularly syndromes of neuropathic etiology: amitriptyline, desipramine, doxepin, imipramine, and clomipramine.
- There is growing documentation of a primary analgesic effect with newer medications such as trazodone, fluoxetine, paroxetine, citalopram, mirtazepine, and sertraline.
- The type of heterocyclic agent prescribed should be based on the degree of sedation desired as well as side-effect profile. Thus, patients with agitation, anxiety, and insomnia will respond better from a sedating heterocyclic such as doxepin, amitriptyline, trazodone, or mirtazepine; those with psychomotor retardation and anergia will often do better on a drug with a more energizing profile, such as nortriptyline, fluoxetine, paroxetine, sertraline, or citalopram.
- Heterocyclics with the earlier mentioned primary autonomic, cardiac, and central nervous side effects may be problematic for older patients with heart disease, glaucoma, or cognitive impairment. Therefore, serotonergic medications may be preferable in this age group, as well as in patients who have a particularly refractory reaction to a previously tried heterocyclic (e.g., increased appetite, intolerable dry mouth, or sedation).
- Heterocyclic antidepressants have also been found to be useful adjuncts to narcotic analgesics in the treatment of chronic pain. Patients on such a combined regimen will tend to tolerate a lower level of narcotic maintenance dosage, without dependence or abuse. Moreover, certain pain syndromes previously refractory to narcotic medication alone may be more responsive to such combined medication.

Finally, many times it is useful to monitor clinical response of an antidepressant medication regimen by drawing blood levels. Although this is not essential for the safe and effective administration of such medications, they can prove useful in the following situations: when an older or more medically complicated patient is being treated; when the clinical response of the patient appears to be ambiguous, raising questions of absorption or patient compliance; and when a medication with a therapeutic window is being prescribed (e.g., imipramine).

Anticonvulsants

It is surprising that certain anticonvulsant agents have been found to be effective in treating chronic pain of neurogenic origin. These include pain syndromes such as migraine headaches, trigeminal neuralgia, diabetic neuropathy, and central thalamic pain syndrome. This is because the patho-physiologic etiology of epilepsy and deafferentation (the elimination or interruption of afferent nerve impulses) pain are quite similar, and such agents stabilize the hyperexcitable neuromembranes of pain-transmitting cells and reduce the repetitive discharge of stimulated second-order neurons (Polatin & Gajraj, 2002). With these drugs, patients are initially started at a low dose and then titrated upward at set intervals, with appropriate monitoring of therapeutic response and emergence of side effects. Blood levels need to be checked periodically, and the total daily dose depends on the therapeutic response or any intolerable side effects. Such side effects can be severe in certain patients, thereby limiting the usefulness of these medications. They may include central nervous system symptoms, such as ataxia (failure or irregularity of muscle coordination), slurred speech, confusion, and drowsiness; gastrointestinal effects, such as nausea and consti-pation; the potential risk of hepatitis or liver damage; and possible anemia and bone marrow suppression. Thus, again, these patients need to be moni-tored carefully, with a full medical evaluation conducted prior to the initia-tion of such a medication regimen. Table 8.3 lists some of the commonly used anticonvulsant medications.

Muscle Relaxants

The term *muscle relaxants* is actually a misnomer, because such agents act directly on the central nervous system to treat muscle spasms and have no actual peripheral action on tight muscles (Polatin & Gajraj, 2002). They can be quite useful in the early treatment of acute musculoskeletal pain. However, they have little therapeutic benefit for chronic pain because they have addictive potential and are associated with a withdrawal syndrome. The one exception is Baclofen, which has been found to be useful in relieving the pain associated with trigeminal neuralgia (pain and numbness of facial structures caused by trigeminal nerve problems) as well as controlling other chronic neuropathic pain syndromes. However, Baclofen too is associated with side effects such as ataxia, confusion, drowsiness, and gastric distress. Clinicians should also be aware of the fact that, after prolonged use of

TABLE 8.3
Anticonvulsants Commonly Used for Chronic Pain and Their Dosage Levels

Drug	Dosage level (mg/day)
Diphenyldantoin (Dilantin)	150–400 (300 average)
Carbamazepine (Tegretol)	100–1600 (400–600 average)
Clonazepam (Klonopin)	1.5–6.0
Valproic acid (Depakene)	250–1000
Gabapentin (Neurontin)	300–3600
Topiramate (Topamax)	25–400
Leutiracetom (Keppra)	500–3000
Tragabine (Gabitril)	2–16
Oxcarbazepine (Trileptal)	600–2400
Lamotrigine (Lamictal)	50–250
Felbamate (Felbatol)	400–3600
Zonisamide (Zonegran)	100–600

Note. Brand names are in parentheses. From "Integration of Pharmacotherapy With Psychological Treatment of Chronic Pain," by P. B. Polatin and N. M. Gajraj, in *Psychological Approaches to Pain Management: A Practitioner's Handbook* (2nd ed., pp. 276–298), edited by D. C. Turk and R. J. Gatchel, 2002, New York: Guilford Press. Copyright 2002 by Guilford Press. Adapted with permission.

this drug, it will need to be tapered off slowly in order to avoid anxiety, hallucinations, and tachycardia.

Anti-Anxiety and Sedative Agents

These medications can be quite useful in treating the noxious, nociceptive effect in acute pain by decreasing the emotional response to it as well as to treat the secondary emotional distress symptoms in chronic-pain patients. The *benzodiazepines* are the major class of such psychotropics used to control anxiety and insomnia in chronic pain. They are also very frequently used in acute pain to decrease muscle spasms or to reduce anticipatory anxiety prior to some critical procedure. There is an array of benzodiazepines that are useful for the short-term treatment of anxiety: Ativan, Librium, Valium, Centrax, Serax, Tranxene, and Xanax. They should be used over a period of a few weeks or months to control the initial symptoms, in coordination with other biopsychosocial interventions. They should then be tapered slowly as the patients stabilize with the use of nonpharmacological treatments such as stress management or other cognitive–behavioral treatment techniques. One can often expect certain side effects, such as drowsiness or ataxia. Moreover, because these medications have an addictive potential (with the risk of tolerance or dependence), they should be used cautiously in patients with either a history of drug abuse or some predisposing psychopathology, which may lead to drug abuse (e.g., current substance abuse disorder, antisocial personality disorder, etc.). Clinicians should also keep in mind that there is a withdrawal syndrome that will require a tapering dosage under careful medical supervision.

Neuroleptics

Neuroleptics are also called *antipsychotic agents* or *major tranquilizers*. Such medications have a potent impact on psychotic behavior and agitation, and they can control chronic-pain syndromes (Polatin & Gajraj, 2002). These agents, though, have significant side effects, including various movement disorders, sedation, and possible cardiac toxicity. Moreover, *tardive dyskinesia* (later onset of impairment of voluntary movements) may pose a significant risk for the long-term continuous use of neuroleptics. With this in mind, along with the lack of solid evidence for a significant effect on chronic-pain states, the use of neuroleptics in chronic pain is limited unless a psychosis or a volatile, disruptive personality disorder requires their usage by specific psychopharmacological guidelines. Some of the commonly used neuroleptics include the following: Thorazine, Mellaril, Stelazine, Haldol, Navane, Risperdal, Seroquel, and Zyprex. The general criteria for their use are (a) when all other anti-anxiety and sedative agents do not have an impact on the patient's emotional distress and (b) there are symptoms of psychosis or disruptive personality disorders.

Other Pharmacotherapeutic Methods

It should also be noted that, to increase the analgesic effectiveness of either non-narcotic analgesics or the opioids, several types of medications have been used with chronic-pain patients (Polatin & Gajraj, 2002). Many peripheral analgesics are also now available (Argoff, Benoist, Brzusek, Figueroa, & Gimbel, 2002). These *adjuvant* agents include the previously discussed antidepressants, neuroleptics, and anticonvulsants often used with chronic pain. Other adjuvant agents include the following:

- Caffeine, which has often been used to enhance NSAID analgesia and shortens the time-of-onset effect.
- Neuroleptics, which sometimes have an enhancing effect on opioid analgesia.
- The use of antihistamines along with opioid therapy in chronic-pain patients, which often allows the use a lower dose narcotic as well as providing additional sedation.
- Psychostimulants, such as Ritalin and Dextroamphetamine, which sometimes augment narcotic analgesia as well as counteract the sedation effects seen with the use of opioids. However, there is a risk of central nervous system toxicity and addiction

with the use of these agents; they therefore must be monitored carefully.

- There are now also certain topical agents available, such as eutectic mixture of local anesthetics cream (a mixture of lidocaine and prilocaine), which can be used to treat postherpetic neuralgia and scar pain. In addition, a topical 5% lidocaine agent (Lidoderm) has also been demonstrated to relieve postherpetic neuralgia pain. Also, Capsaicin cream has been found to be useful in the treatment of neuropathic pain conditions, such as diabetic neuropathy pain; however, it is limited because of side effects such as burning and localized itching and rash. Overall, recent advances in the understanding of the underlying mechanisms, as well as the clinical utility, of topical analgesics have provided some exciting new therapeutic options for patients with acute or chronic pain. A more thorough review of these agents was presented by Argoff and colleagues (2002).

Drug Interaction Effects

A great many drugs have been reviewed thus far that are commonly used with patients suffering from pain. Managing the physical and psychological complaints of patients, especially those of patients with chronic pain, is often a complex task that frequently requires multiple medications. These may include narcotics, muscle relaxants, anticonvulsants, NSAIDs, antidepressants, anxiolytics, neuroleptics, sedatives, and other agents. The challenge of medication management for chronic pain is to provide symptom relief while avoiding individual or cumulative side effects or toxicities. Many of these agents have the potential to cause central nervous system depression as manifested by oversedation, loss of cognitive facility, demotivation, anergia, and even emotional depression. The combination of two or more of these agents together will have cumulatively much more potential for central nervous system depression. Therefore, clinicians must maintain close surveillance of the mental status and current functional level of patients who are under medication management. The utility of various medications in a regimen should periodically be evaluated, and medications that are not effective should be discontinued before new ones are started. Unfortunately, it is all too frequently the case that a pain patient goes from physician to physician, each one of whom adds more medication without tapering any of the previously used agents. Even nonphysician clinicians should be aware of adverse effects, side effects, and interactions of medications used to treat the various symptoms of chronic pain. Such information may be available in certain standard references that are updated annually, such as the *Physicians' Desk Reference* and *The Handbook of Adverse Drug Interactions*, pub-

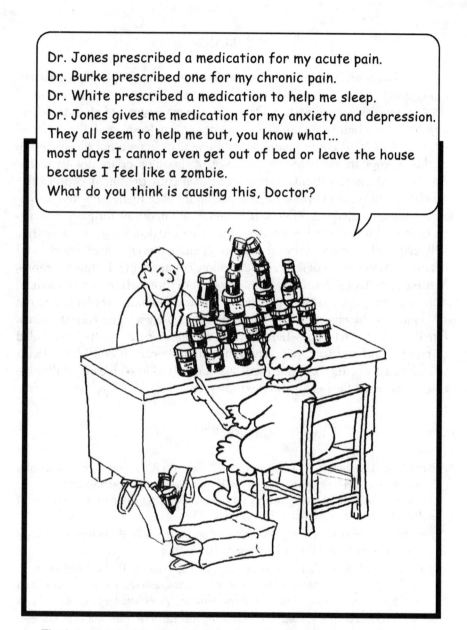

The importance of carefully documenting all medications being taken by a patient in order to prevent unwanted side effects and adverse interactions.

lished by the Medical Letter on Drugs and Therapeutics. There is also a more frequently updated program of pharmaceutical information, including the capability of listing up to 30 individual drugs for a multicheck of interactive side effects, available to be downloaded from www.epocrates.com. This can be used through either a computer or a personal digital assistant (PDA).

SUMMARY

As I have reviewed, it is fortunate that there is a panoply of pharmaceutical agents that may be used in the treatment of pain and the emotional distress often associated with it. Of course, the major goals of pharmacotherapy in comprehensive pain management are analgesia and the relief of emotional distress. Often, many general practitioners are not always aware of the appropriate medications to use or of the appropriate dosage levels. As a consequence, patients may present at a pain treatment center on a number of different pharmacological agents that are ineffective and associated with unwanted side effects. It is therefore important for pain management specialists to be acutely aware of pharmacological agents because they will frequently have to unravel a range of inappropriate medications, and begin a new pharmacological regimen, before commencing the more comprehensive pain management program. For a more thorough review of medications used for pain and their mechanisms of analgesia, the reader is referred to "Pain and Mechanisms of Analgesia" (http://www.sigma-aldridh.com). Finally, as was discussed, when all pain management attempts have failed to relieve pain and to regain function, palliative care is considered (with opioids usually being the prime medication involved in such care). Palliative care is discussed further in the next chapter.

REFERENCES

Adams, L. L., Gatchel, R. J., Robinson, R. C., Polatin, P. P., Gajraj, N., Deschner, M., et al. (2004). Development of a self-report screening instrument for assessing potential opioid medication misuse in chronic pain patients. *Journal of Pain and Symptom Management, 27*, 440–459.

American Pain Society. (1992). *Principles of analgesic use in the treatment of acute pain and cancer pain* (3rd ed.). Skokie, IL: Author.

Argoff, C. E., Benoist, J. L., Brzusek, D. A., Figueroa, J. P., & Gimbel, J. S. (2002, August). Clinical advances in pain management: Targeted peripheral analgesics. [Spec. supp. Endo Pharmaceuticals]. *Anesthesiology News*, 1–12.

Cole, B. E. (2002, January/February). Mastering medications. *Practical Pain Management*, 27–31.

Cole, B. E. (2003). Balancing pain management and professional risk. *Practical Pain Management, 3*, 23–29.

Cooper, J., Czechowicz, D., Peterson, R., & Molinan, S. (1992). Prescription drug diversion control and medical practice. *Journal of the American Medical Association, 268*, 1306–1310.

Dersh, J., Polatin, P., & Gatchel, R. (2002). Chronic pain and psychopathology: Research findings and theoretical considerations. *Psychosomatic Medicine, 64*, 773–786.

Harden, R. N. (2002). Chronic opioid therapy: Another reappraisal. *APS Bulletin, 12*, 1–12.

Hochman, J., Anderson, A. V., & Tennant, F. (2003, January/February). Antidepressants in pain treatment. *Practical Pain Management*, 12–14.

Jamison, R. N. (2002). Addiction and pain assessment and treatment issues. *Clinical Journal of Pain, 18*(Suppl.).

Julien, R. M. (1981). *A primer of drug action* (3rd ed.). New York: Freeman.

Liaison Committee on Pain and Addiction. (2001). *Definitions related to the use of opioids for the treatment of pain: A consensus document from the American Academy of Pain Medicine, the American Pain Society, and the American Society of Addiction Medicine*. Retrieved February 27, 2003, from http://www.ampainsoc. org/advocacy/opioids2.htm

National Center for Health Statistics. (1998). *National Ambulatory Medical Care Survey, 1998*. Washington, DC: U.S. Department of Health and Human Services.

Oliver, R. L., & Taylor, A. (2003, March/April). Chronic opioid rules. *Practical Pain Management*, 30–36.

Polatin, P. B., & Gajraj, N. M. (2002). Integration of pharmacotherapy with psychological treatment of chronic pain. In D. C. Turk & R. J. Gatchel (Eds.), *Psychological approaches to pain management: A practitioner's handbook* (2nd ed., pp. 276–298). New York: Guilford Press.

Portenoy, R., & Foley, K. (1986). Chronic use of opioid analgesics in nonmalignant pain: Report of 38 cases. *Pain, 25*, 171–186.

Schappert, S. M. (1998). Ambulatory care visits to physicians' offices, hospital outpatient departments, and emergency departments: United States, 1996. *Vital and Health Statistics, Series 13*(134), 1–80.

Shanti, B. F., Tan, G., & Shenaq, S. A. (2001, November/December). Opioid rotation: Mechanisms, concepts and benefits. *Practical Pain Management*, 8–11.

Turk, D. C. (in press). Pain management. In C. Spielberger (Ed.), *Encyclopedia of applied psychology*. San Diego, CA: Academic Press.

Twycross, R. (1994). Opioids. In P. Wall & R. Melzack (Eds.), *Textbook of pain* (pp. 325–370). New York: Churchill Livingstone.

APPENDIX 8.1

Recommended Readings

Cole, B. E. (2002, January/February). Mastering medications. *Practical Pain Management, 27–31.*

Polatin, P. B., & Gajraj, N. M. (2002). Integration of pharmacotherapy with psychological treatment of chronic pain. In D. C. Turk & R. J. Gatchel (Eds.), *Psychological approaches to pain management: A practitioner's handbook* (2nd ed., pp. 276–298). New York: Guilford Press.

http://www.epocrates.com

APPENDIX 8.2

Medication Responsibility Agreement

Medications are very useful; however, controlled substance medications (i.e., narcotics) have a high potential for misuse and therefore are closely controlled by local, state, and federal agencies. My physician is prescribing medications, some of which may be controlled substances, to help manage pain and lead to improved function; therefore, I agree to the following conditions:

1. I am responsible for the medications prescribed to me and for keeping track of the amount remaining.
2. Medication refills:
   - **Call the pharmacist 3–5 days before** a refill is due. The pharmacist will contact the Pain Center to initiate the refill. Allow at least 2 working days for the Pain Center to authorize the refill.
   - If there are no more refills, call to schedule an appointment with the prescribing physician. **It is my responsibility to make sure I have an appointment scheduled before the time that I will run out of medication.**
   - **Refills will not be made** if "I run out early," "lose my prescription," or "spill or misplace my medication."
   - **Refills will not be made** on an "emergency" basis. It is my responsibility to keep track of the amount of medication I have left.
3. As part of the Interdisciplinary Pain Management Program, I will be required to attend all components of the treatment plan, developed by me and my treatment team, in order that I receive maximum benefit and opportunity for improvement. I understand that the main treatment goal is to reduce pain and to improve my ability to function and/or work. In consideration of this goal, and the fact that I am being given a potent

medication to help me reach my goal, I agree to help myself by the following better health habits (i.e., exercise, weight control, and avoidance of excessive tobacco and alcohol use). If I fail to participate in all components of the treatment plan, it may result in termination from the program and discontinuance of medication refills.

4. I agree to comply with random urine, blood, or breath testing documenting the proper use of my medication as well as confirming compliance. I understand that driving a motor vehicle may not be allowed while taking controlled substance medications and that it is my responsibility to comply with the laws of the state while taking the prescribed medications.

5. I understand that if I violate any of the above conditions, my prescriptions may be terminated immediately. If the violation involves obtaining the controlled substance from another individual or the concomitant use of nonprescribed illicit (illegal) drugs, I may also be reported to all of my physicians, medical facilities, and appropriate authorities.

6. I understand the long-term advantages and disadvantages of chronic narcotic use (if applicable) have yet to be scientifically determined and that my treatment may change at any time. I understand, accept, and agree that there may be unknown risks associated with the long-term use of controlled substances and that my physician will advise me of any advances in this field and will make treatment changes as needed.

I have been fully informed by my physician and the staff regarding psychological dependence (addiction) of controlled substances, which I understand is rare (if relevant to my treatment plan). I know that some individuals may develop a tolerance to the medications, necessitating a dose increase to achieve the desired effect, and that there is a risk of becoming physically dependent on the medication. This will occur if I am on the medication for several weeks. Therefore, when I need to stop taking the medication, I must do it slowly under medical direction, or I may suffer withdrawal symptoms.

I have read this agreement and the same has been explained to me by my physician or his nurse. In addition, I fully understand the consequences of violating this agreement.

Patient Signature:

——————————————————————— Date ——————————

Witness Signature:

——————————————————————— Date ——————————

APPENDIX 8.3

Example Medication Refill Policy

- If you miss your doctor's appointment, you will not be able to call in and have your prescription filled.
- Please schedule your next doctor's appointment before leaving the office today.
- To receive your prescription, you have to keep your doctor's appointment.
- If you miss a doctor's appointment, and you would like to have your prescription refilled, you must come back to this office as a "walk-in" patient to see the doctor. In this case, please let the front desk know that you are a walk-in for a medication check.
- Also, before you come in, please check the label on your prescription bottle to see **if you have any refills left,** or ask your pharmacy to check their hard copy to see that *all* refills have been used.

Thank you.

APPENDIX 8.4

Pain Medication Questionnaire

NAME: _____

In order to develop the best treatment plan for you, we want to understand your thoughts, needs and experiences related to pain medication. Please read each statement below and indicate how much it applies to you by marking your response with an "X" anywhere on the line below it.

1) I believe I am receiving enough medication to relieve my pain.

Disagree	Somewhat Disagree	Neutral	Somewhat Agree	Agree

2) My doctor spends enough time talking to me about my pain medication during appointments.

Disagree	Somewhat Disagree	Neutral	Somewhat Agree	Agree

3) I believe I would feel better with a higher dosage of my pain medication.

Disagree	Somewhat Disagree	Neutral	Somewhat Agree	Agree

4) In the past, I have had some difficulty getting the medication I need from my doctor(s).

| Disagree | Somewhat Disagree | Neutral | Somewhat Agree | Agree |

5) I wouldn't mind quitting my current pain medication and trying a new one, if my doctor recommends it.

| Disagree | Somewhat Disagree | Neutral | Somewhat Agree | Agree |

6) I have clear preferences about the type of pain medication I need.

| Disagree | Somewhat Disagree | Neutral | Somewhat Agree | Agree |

7) Family members seem to think that I may be too dependent on my pain medication.

| Disagree | Somewhat Disagree | Neutral | Somewhat Agree | Agree |

8) It is important to me to try ways of managing my pain in addition to the medication (*such as relaxation, biofeedback, physical therpay, TENS unit, etc.*)

| Disagree | Somewhat Disagree | Neutral | Somewhat Agree | Agree |

9) At times, I take pain medication when I feel anxious and sad, or when I need help sleeping.

| Never | Occasionally | Sometimes | Often | Always |

10) At times, I drink alcohol to help control my pain.

| Never | Occasionally | Sometimes | Often | Always |

11) My pain medication makes it hard for me to think clearly sometimes.

| Never | Occasionally | Sometimes | Often | Always |

12) I find it necessary to go to the emergency room to get treatment for my pain.

| Never | Occasionally | Sometimes | Often | Always |

13) My pain medication makes me nauseated and constipated sometimes.

| Never | Occasionally | Sometimes | Often | Always |

14) At times, I need to borrow pain medication from friends or family to get relief.

Never	Occasionally	Sometimes	Often	Always

15) I get pain medication from more than one doctor in order to have enough medication for my pain.

Never	Occasionally	Sometimes	Often	Always

16) At times, I think I may be too dependent on my pain medication.

Never	Occasionally	Sometimes	Often	Always

17) To help me out, family members have obtained pain medications for me from their own doctors.

Never	Occasionally	Sometimes	Often	Always

18) At times, I need to take pain medication more often than it is prescribed in order to relieve my pain.

Never	Occasionally	Sometimes	Often	Always

19) I save any unused pain medication I have in case I need it later.

Never	Occasionally	Sometimes	Often	Always

20) I find it helpful to call my doctor or clinic to talk about how my pain medication is working.

Never	Occasionally	Sometimes	Often	Always

21) At times, I run out of pain medication early and have to call my doctor for refills.

Never	Occasionally	Sometimes	Often	Always

22) I find it useful to take additional medications (such as sedatives) to help my pain medication work better.

Never	Occasionally	Sometimes	Often	Always

23) How many painful conditions (injured body parts or illnesses) do you have?

1 painful condition	2 painful conditions	3 painful conditions	4 painful conditions	5+ painful conditions

24) How many times in the past <u>year</u> have you asked your doctor to increase your prescribed dosage of pain medication in order to get relief?

Never	1 time	2 times	3 times	4+ times

25) How many times in the past <u>year</u> have you run out of pain medication early and had to request an early refill?

Never	1 time	2 times	3 times	4+ times

26) How many times in the past <u>year</u> have you accidentally misplaced your prescription for pain medication and had to ask for another?

Never	1 time	2 times	3 times	4+ times

9

THE ROLE OF PALLIATIVE CARE METHODS IN PAIN MANAGEMENT

What we call pleasure, and rightly so, is the absence of all pain.
—Cicero
Among the remedies which it has pleased Almighty God to give man
to relieve his sufferings, none is so universal and so efficacious as opium.
—Sydenham (see Taylor, 1965)

As Lipman (2002) pointed out, pain management and palliative care have grown in parallel in the United States in recent years. Many pain specialists consider palliative care as the final phase of treatment of pain, after all other approaches have been attempted or ruled out and found to be ineffective in helping a patient to regain function or experience some significant degree of relief from unremitting pain. Tennant, Liu, and Hermann (2002) delineated some of the common characteristics of these patients:

- The pain is unremitting and excruciating.
- The patient is bed-, chair-, or housebound when not on opioid treatment.
- The pain is reducing sleep and food intake.
- The patient may be experiencing confusion, attention deficits, depression, and suicidal ideation.
- The underlying cause of the pain is incurable or nonremovable and has failed to respond to all other pain treatment efforts.
- There is evidence of a great deal of stress due to the pain (e.g., elevated heart rate, blood pressure, and hormonal irregularities).

The primary goal of intervention at this stage is to provide some comfort to the patient in a cost-effective manner while maintaining maximum capacity for physical functioning. It is expected that, after and during palliative care treatment, these patients will experience some decrease in unremitting pain symptoms, with partial return to adaptive functioning. Moreover, another goal is that these patients will decrease their dependence on financial or health benefits and return to normalized activities of daily living.

In this chapter, I review the various palliative care modalities now available for pain management. Such care originally received the most attention in the area of cancer pain, where the World Health Organization Expert Committee (1990) defined it as follows:

> The active total care of patients whose disease is not responsive to curative treatment. Control of pain, of other symptoms, and of psychological, social and spiritual problems, is paramount. The goal of palliative care is the achievement of the best quality of life for patients and their families. Many aspects of palliative care are also applicable earlier in the course of the illness in conjunction with anti-cancer treatment. (p. 28)

In this context, Carney and Meier (2000) view palliative care as an interdisciplinary team endeavor in which physicians, nurses, psychologists, and other health care professionals are involved in the treatment process. Key elements include providing psychosocial and spiritual support, assuring physical comfort to both the patient and his or her family, and providing coordinated services across different care sites when needed. Palliative care itself originated in London in 1967 when Dame Cicely Saunders established Saint Christopher's Hospice. Even though palliative care is a well-established medical subspecialty in major academic centers in the United Kingdom, Canada, and Australia, as well as several other countries, it is still struggling to gain a solid foundation in the United States (Garvin, 1999).

Of course, palliative care may be beneficial not only with cancer pain but also with unremitting chronic-pain syndromes. In this chapter, I review various modalities, such as injection procedures, spinal cord stimulators, and implanted morphine pumps. Of course, as I pointed out in the last chapter, there is a clinical bias against palliative care (when opioids are prescribed), which is driven by legal considerations and the fear of abuse problems. Fortunately, however, this clinical bias is beginning to change somewhat (Joint Commission on Accreditation of Healthcare Organizations, 2000). Indeed, there was a major public outcry for the humane treatment of patients with chronic nonmalignant pain including long-term maintenance from narcotics. For example, some states have drafted principles of the responsible professional practice for such use of opioids in chronic-pain patients. These recommendations include the following: a patient history;

physical examination; informed consent from the patient; a formulated treatment plan; periodic review of the patient's case; consultation whenever necessary; accurate record keeping; and strict compliance with controlled-substances regulations. However, the overuse of opioids for any or all pain syndromes is being challenged, and the pendulum is swinging toward the moderate-use position (Harden, 2002).

Lipman (2002) appropriately noted that palliative care usually requires a different philosophical approach from curative care when treating patients with pain. He presented a summary of the contrasts between the philosophical constructs for these two approaches (see Exhibit 9.1).

PALLIATIVE CARE TREATMENT MODALITIES

Deschner and Polatin (2000) reviewed the types of treatment that are consistent with palliative care, which include the following:

- Medical maintenance procedures for episodic pain.
- Instruction in fitness maintenance programs.
- Relaxation training, coping, and stress management techniques.
- Injection procedures, such as peripheral and sympathetic nerve blocks to reduce the transmission from pain sites and used for diagnosable and therapeutic purposes.
- Cognitive–behavioral programs.
- Limited passive modalities, such as massage and transcutaneous electrical nerve stimulation.
- The use of secondary, tertiary, or surgical procedures that may be tried or repeated for severe recurrence of pain.
- Socioeconomic interventions, such as vocational and rehabilitation and disability case management, to resolve any outstanding injury-related financial award.
- For control of intractable pain, external devices, such as a spinal cord stimulator and analgesic pumps may be tried, as well as denervation procedures or long-term opioid maintenance.

I now review some of the approaches in the last of the above categories, because they are being increasingly used today.

Injection Procedures

Injections have become common procedures in pain management, and they may be performed at various anatomic sites. Moreover, they may be used as a therapeutic modality, as well as diagnostically to help identify

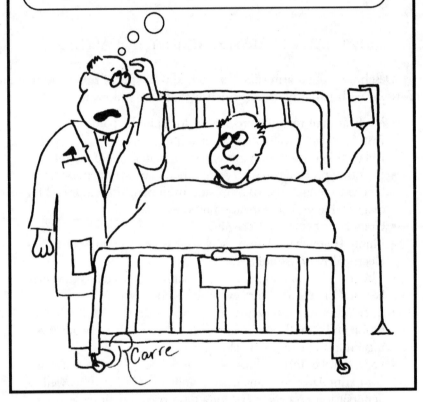

The dilemma often faced by health care professionals when faced with the need to prescribe more narcotics in order to reduce a patient's pain.

potential pain generators. Prognostically, they may be helpful in predicting the outcome of more invasive procedures. Because pain management specialists will often encounter injection procedures performed in a patient's medical record, it is useful to be aware of what they are used for. These procedures are summarized in Exhibit 9.2. Noe, Gajraj, and Vakharia (2000) provided a more extensive review of such procedures.

EXHIBIT 9.1
Philosophical Constructs for Cure-Focused Care and Palliative Care

Cure-Focused Care	Palliative Care
Cure is the goal	Symptom control is the goal
Analytical and rationalistic	Subjective
Based on diagnoses	Based on symptoms
Scientific and biomedical	Humanistic and personal
Aimed at disease process	Aimed at comfort
Views patients as parts	Views patient as whole
Based on "hard" sciences	Based on "soft" social sciences
Impersonal care	Individualized care
Hierarchical	Interdisciplinary
Death is seen as failure	Death is accepted as normal

Note. From "Pain Management and Palliative Care," by A. G. Lipman, 2002, *APS Bulletin, 12,* pp. 3–17. Copyright 2002 by American Pain Society. Reprinted with permission.

Spinal Cord Stimulators

During the past decade, there has been an expanding role of spinal cord stimulation as a treatment option for the palliative care of chronic pain. Stimulated by Melzack and Wall's (1965) *gate-control theory of pain,* which I reviewed in chapter 1 and which proposes that the activation of low-threshold afferent nerve fibers decreases the response of dorsal horn neurons to unmyelinated nociceptors (thereby "closing the gate" to pain transmission from the spinal cord), a number of clinical applications of this theory have been developed. Shealy, Mortimer, and Rewick (1967) were the first to apply this when they stimulated the dorsal columns for the treatment of chronic, intractable pain. Since that time, implantable dorsal column stimulation (i.e., spinal cord stimulation [SCS]) was developed to treat a wide variety of pain syndromes. As Cameron and Elliott (2002) noted, since the time that the SCS procedure was first inspired by the gate-control theory, its effectiveness is now also linked to a number of other mechanisms, such as the activation of spinal pain inhibitory circuits as well as regional blood flow to various regions at the cerebral level.

In SCS, electrodes for the stimulators are inserted through an epidural needle, usually with the use of local anesthesia. These electrodes are then attached to a passive receiving device or a battery-powered stimulator. Once the optimal stimulating parameters have been identified, patients usually control the strength and duration of the stimulation. It should also be noted that peripheral nerve stimulation can be administered through cuff electrodes that are placed around a peripheral nerve at the area of the injury site.

SCS has frequently been used for many patients with failed back surgery syndrome as an alternative to reoperation (e.g., North, Kidd, Zahurak, James, & Long, 1993). In addition, it has been used to treat reflex sympathetic

EXHIBIT 9.2
Summary of Common Injection Procedures

Peripheral nerve blocks are often used as a diagnostic method with peripheral nerve entrapment conditions, especially in the upper extremities.

Selective nerve root blocks are frequently used with patients previously treated with surgery as a diagnostic procedure. These include the following: medial branch blocks, continuous brachial plexus blocks, dorsal root ganglion blocks, sympathetic nerve blocks, cervical sympathetic blocks, thoracic sympathetic blocks, lumbar sympathetic blocks, and piriformis injections; muscle blocks.

Joint injections involve intra-articular injections with a corticosteroid or a local anesthetic for most joints. These include sacroiliac joint injections and facet blocks (e.g., lumbar facet and cervical facet injections).

Bursa injections are for common bursae in the hip, knee, hindfoot, and the coronal section of the shoulder.

Tendon injections are commonly used for treating tendonitis involving the rotator cuff, biceps, and other tendons.

Triggerpoint and tender-point injections usually involve injecting myofascial trigger-points and fibromyalgia tender points with various substances (most commonly a local anesthetic).

Epidural steroid injections are frequently used for spinal pain involving radicular pain, to reduce nerve root inflammation in conditions such as lumbar disc disease, spinal stenosis, and postlaminectomy syndrome.

Intrathecal Baclofena (lioresal) injections (injections within the sheath of the spinal cord) are used for the spasticity associated with conditions such as spinal cord injury, cerebral palsy, or head injuries when oral medications have been found to be unsuccessful in terms of either efficacy or unwanted side effects.

---

dystrophy, postamputation pain, postherpetic neuralgia, spinal cord injury dysesthesias, and pain associated with multiple sclerosis (Long, 1998). North et al. (1993) reported that, for neuropathic pain, continued pain relief was found in 70% of patients using a multichannel system and in 30% of patients using a single-channel system. Grabow, Tella, and Raja (2003) also reviewed evidence for SCS effectiveness in patients with complex regional pain syndrome who did not respond to more conservative pain management.

Prager and Jacobs (2001) emphasized the importance of accurate diagnosis, with patient selection through a comprehensive biopsychosocial evaluation, if implantable pain therapy is to be successful. Indeed, Nelson and colleagues (1996) delineated the following screening criteria that should be used to *exclude* patients from consideration for SCS implantation:

- active psychosis;
- active suicidality;
- active homicidality;
- untreated or poorly treated major mood disorders, such as major depression;

- an unusually high level of somatization or other somatoform disorders;
- substance abuse disorders;
- unresolved workers' compensation or litigation cases;
- lack of appropriate social support; and
- cognitive defects that compromise adequate reasoning and memory.

Although this patient-screening approach is still somewhat imprecise, and until a more refined screening approach is thoroughly developed, it will undoubtedly make an important contribution to more reliable prediction of response to such treatment. It is important because these criteria reflect potential problems, such as lack of understanding on how to use the device; the internal sensations generated by the device that may be difficult to deal with, especially in patients who are predisposed to somatic delusions; and significant psychosocial problems that will continue to exacerbate pain complaints regardless of medical treatment. These issues will need to be dealt with before one can guarantee any degree of success (Doleys, 2002).

Implanted Morphine Pumps

Another type of implantable pain management modality is *intraspinal therapy*. This involves drugs being delivered through implanted catheters with a subcutaneous injection site, a totally implanted catheter with an implanted reservoir and manual pump, or a totally implanted catheter with an implanted infusion pump. As Prager and Jacobs (2001) indicated, the choice of system used depends on the following: the clear indication for intraspinal therapy; a need for a bolus (i.e., a single high dose) versus continuous infusion; the patient's overall medical status; the patient's ambulatory status and available social support services; the patient's life expectancy; and cost. Prager and Jacobs indicated that a fully implanted pump is economically feasible if the patient's life expectancy is greater than 3 months. Hassenbusch and Portenoy (2000) reviewed physician-practice patterns concerning the long-term use of this modality and concluded that there were wide variations among physicians in its use. Moreover, they emphasized the need for practice guidelines, developed on the basis of methodologically sound research outcomes, combined with input from experienced experts in the field, to develop methods for optimizing pain management with this modality. Bennett (2000) also emphasized the need for more consensus based on evidence-based research as to what compounds or agents are best for this type of therapy. Currently, morphine and bysibacaine appear the most widely used.

Again, just as in the case of the SCS modality, interdisciplinary evaluations of patients need to be the standard of care in this area before patients are considered for this modality. Such patients' prescreening is essential for good therapeutic outcomes with all of these modalities (Gatchel, 2001). Block, Gatchel, Deardorff, and Guyer (2003) presented a useful presurgical psychological screening approach to use with surgical patients, such as those receiving implantable devices, as well as guidelines for pre- and post-surgical treatment.

Use of Opioids for Long-Term Palliative Care

In the last chapter, I discussed the use of opioid therapy in the management of chronic pain as a major means of managing chronic pain that cannot be treated by surgical or conservative treatment. As Robinson, Gatchel, Polatin, Deschner, and Noe (2001) noted, this has created a greater need for physicians to become aware of the appropriate use of such medication. The development of such an awareness is frequently perceived as a daunting task by many physicians, who must decide when it is appropriate to start using opioids for managing chronic pain. One concern mentioned in chapter 8 is the perception of potential addiction or harmful consequences of chronic opioid use. There has actually been some recent patient-initiated litigation against physicians for allegedly causing opioid addiction (Gatchel, 2001). Conversely, with the new guidelines presented by Joint Commission on the Accreditation of Healthcare Organizations, it is now mandated that physicians must actively assist in managing patients' pain if opioids are necessary. This has stimulated the search for a method of determining potential risk factors for opioid misuse in chronic-pain patients in order to evaluate which patient may be safely and appropriately maintained on opioid medication. Potential useful screening evaluations are now being developed (e.g., Adams et al., 2004; Robinson et al., 2001). The one constructed by Adams and colleagues (2004) was presented in Appendix 8.4.

As I have highlighted (Gatchel, 2001), opioid analgesics continue to be the most widely used and effective analgesic class for many acute- and chronic-pain syndromes. Even its use in the management of postoperative and chronic nonmalignant pain is becoming increasingly accepted as a viable option for treatment. With chronic usage, though, patients may develop tolerance to the analgesic effects of these opioids. In response to such problems, laboratory research has been conducted to examine ways of eliminating intolerable side effects and tolerance in a safe manner. A survey of investigations has revealed some impressive data to suggest that opioid analgesia can be enhanced with the addition of N-methyl-D-aspartate antagonists, such as dextromethorphan, or by the use of a concomitant ultra low dose opioid antagonist. The results of these initial studies are quite promising, and they deserve additional follow-up to maximize the potential of this new approach to minimize the negative side effects and tolerance problems often seen in opioid treatment, especially when it is chronic and palliative in nature.

Oliver and Taylor (2003) provided a useful set of rules for prescribing opioids. These rules, along with potential warning signs of abuse, as well as success signs of nonabuse, are presented in Table 9.1.

It is also useful to keep in mind patients who may be at a high risk of misuse or abuse. Relevant variables include the following:

- a past addiction/substance abuse history;
- untreated anxiety and depression;
- personality disorders/dysfunctions, such as oppositional non-compliance
- financial and social problems.

APPROPRIATE PALLIATIVE CARE FOR PATIENTS WITH CANCER PAIN

Because cancer patients represent the largest group of chronic-pain patients in medicine today, and because they are most in need of effective pain control methods, more specific details are provided concerning this patient population (of course, much of this information is also applicable to many unremitting pain conditions in general). Indeed, there are 1.2 million people diagnosed with cancer each year, and 25% of all deaths in the United States are the result of cancer (Chang, 1999). Moreover, investigations have shown that cancer pain is also significantly undertreated, with elderly individuals and members of ethnic minority groups at the greatest risk (Hewitt, 2001). The Alliance of Cancer Pain Initiatives has also noted the following facts: Up to 70% of cancer patients will experience pain during their illness; at least 90% of cancer-related pain can be relieved; 50% to 70% of patients receive inadequate treatment; and surveys indicate that patients fear pain more than they fear dying from the disease (see http://www.aacpi.wisc.edu).

Cancer pain is not limited to pain caused by the disease itself; pain also is associated with the treatment of cancer (i.e., pain from surgery, chemotherapy, and radiation treatment). Most patients experiencing cancer pain also develop concurrent physical and psychosocial symptoms, such as fatigue, psychological distress, and depression. This again emphasizes the importance of a thorough biopsychosocial assessment when managing cancer pain.

The World Health Organization's cancer pain relief program has estimated that 5 million people worldwide experience cancer pain on a daily

TABLE 9.1
Summary of Rules of Opioid Prescribing

	Rule	Warning signs	Success
1	Single physician Single pharmacy	• Self-pay (patient is using insurance with another physician) • No referring physician (patient has another physician) • Out of town (patient has another physician in his or her hometown) • Obtaining opioids or other narcotics from other physicians or from the street	No signs of another doctor or pharmacy
2	Thorough history and physical, including documentation	• Hysterical or overrated pain scale • Psychological abnormalities • Lack of other chronic pain indicators • Normal or hysterical physical examination • Normal tests	• Realistic pain scale • Level pain scale • Objective findings • Documentation of disorder that correlates with level of pain
3	Urine drug screen	• Negative drug screen for prescribing drug • Positive drug screen for other opioids or illicit drugs	Positive for prescribed drug only
4	Make appropriate consults	• Patient is accusatory of other physicians • Patient refuses referrals, consults, or testing	• Patient agrees to timely consults • Patient follows up with ongoing psychological/ psychiatric treatment
5	Monthly visits	• Frequent phone calls • Early refills • Stories • No significant improvement in pain or function with dose increases from month to month • Wide ranging pain scale • Office visits overly devoted to drug	• Pain decreases in response to dose or proportional to dose escalation • Improvements should be seen month to month until a tolerable level of pain is reached
6	Comorbid conditions treated	Fatigue, anxiety, depression, insomnia, and sexual dysfunction continues	• Comorbid conditions improve • Function improves • Support of a relative or friend in process of improving pain/ function

(continues)

TABLE 9.1 *(Continued)*

	Rule	Warning signs	Success
7	A signed agreement	• Concurrent use of other illicit drugs or addictive drugs • Nonadherence to contract rules • Acceleration of drug use other than prescribed	Follows rules
8	Use long-acting opioids for chronic pain and short-acting opioids for breakthrough pain	• Inconsistent opioid response • Intolerant of Duragesic patch • Preference for short-acting opioids • Intolerance or dislike of other opioids except patient's drug of choice	• Function and/or activity increased significantly • Preference for long-acting opioids • Level pain scale
9	Maximum effective dose	• Tolerated dose is infinite • Overwhelming concern for drug • Short-acting opioids work better than long-acting opioids at equivalent doses • Never happy with any dose and always wanting dose escalation • Pain level never changes despite dose change	• Patient accepts that pain level will never be zero • Equianalgesic action across long-acting opioids • Rational use of breakthrough medication
10	Avoid opioids in drug abusers	History of illicit drugs, alcohol abuse, and prescription drug abuse	No history or evidence of substance abuse

Note. From "Chronic Opioid Rules," by R. L. Oliver and A. Taylor, in *Practical Pain Management,* March/April 2003, pp. 30–36. Copyright 2003 by Practical Pain Management. Reprinted with permission.

basis, with one in four dying from it without any relief from pain (Chang, 1999). To assist physicians in treating cancer patients, the World Health Organization has developed a three-step analgesic ladder (Hewitt, 2001):

1. *Step 1*, intended to treat mild pain, recommends the use of a nonopioid analgesic, such as Motrin, Vioxx, or Tylenol.
2. *Step 2*, for moderate pain, recommends the use of weak opioids, such as Tylenol 3 (Tylenol with codeine) and Darvocet.
3. *Step 3* is intended for treatment of severe pain, and it is recommended that the most powerful opioids, such as morphine and Dilaudid, be used.

Adjuvant therapy with medications from the lower steps may also be used in Steps 2 and 3. It is also recommended that physicians be flexible in their treatment regimens, because it is well documented that individuals respond quite differently to various medications. It should also be kept in mind that, as discussed in the last chapter, there are different routes of administration of medications (e.g., oral, sublingual, intravenous, etc.). For patients experiencing side effects from opioids, switching the delivery and type of pharmaceutical can often provide relief. For all patients, regular pain assessment is mandatory. Some key points to remember are the following:

- Use the same pain rating scales at pre- and post-intervention.
- Initially, assess the pain on administration and at least every 4 hours, or more frequently.
- Collect pre- and post-intervention ratings of pain to evaluate effectiveness.
- Use *consistent documentation* methods.

Quite often, the final, optimal pain regimen for a particular patient is established only after several rounds of trial and error. A pain management specialist also needs to be ready to work closely with the medical oncologist, who assumes the primary role of physician responsible for the provision and coordination of cancer care. This may be extremely challenging and demands a wide range of clinical and interpersonal skills (Cherny & Catane, 1996).

The Need for Multiple Treatment Modalities

As with other forms of chronic pain management, multiple treatment modalities, incorporating nonpharmacologic therapies into pain management plans, should always be considered. These might include methods such as acupuncture, biofeedback, electric nerve stimulation, massage, hypnosis, and exercise (Abraham & Snyder, 2001). Indeed, these additional therapies are quite beneficial in that they relieve some of the anxiety and fear that can often exacerbate pain in patients. Again, incorporating pain management into a broad interdisciplinary treatment approach should be the major goal in treatment programs with cancer patients experiencing pain. In fact, the American Society of Anesthesiologists Task Force on Pain Management (1996) developed guidelines for cancer pain management that are interdisciplinary in nature. The guidelines outline six essential features for a comprehensive biopsychosocial evaluation: (a) history taking, (b) physical examination, (c) psychosocial evaluation, (d) impression and differential diagnoses, (e) diagnostic evaluation, and (f) a treatment plan. Moreover, the task force further recommended that three fundamental concepts be embraced for the longitudinal monitoring of pain: (a) the patient's self-report of pain on a 0-to-10 rating scale; (b) specification of one self-report should be obtained at regular intervals; and (c) documentation when there is either new pain, a change in pattern or intensity of pain, or when a major therapeutic intervention is performed. This task force report also concluded that multidisciplinary specialists resulted in effective analgesia and improved other outcomes for cancer pain patients. It also recommended psychosocial intervention for the management of cancer pain by including pain diaries, biofeedback, hypnosis, relaxation training, psychotherapy, and cognitive–behavioral therapy, all of which have been shown to improve analgesia and patients' quality of life. Indeed, in a recent meta-analysis of social cognitive therapy with cancer patients, Graves (2003) concluded that such treatment maximizes improvement in the overall quality of life in adult cancer patients.

Young and Ades (2001) provided an appropriate summary of cancer pain management to end this discussion:

> The goal of cancer pain therapy is to provide the maximum relief to the patient with minimum side effects. Success of effective pain management depends on an accurate assessment of the patient's pain. Effective treatment techniques and treatment guidelines are now widely available which allow clinicians to provide pain relief for the vast majority of patients with cancer. However, like all areas of medicine there is sometimes a need to refer patients to specialists if the complexity of pain management required exceeds the physician's experience. (p. 13)

SUICIDE RISK IN PATIENTS WITH UNREMITTING CHRONIC PAIN AND/OR CANCER

As Crichton and Morley (2002) noted, the great fear of pain and a painful death is quite common in patients with cancer, as well as in patients with other unremitting chronic-pain syndromes. Fortunately, with the advent of more effective pain management techniques, severe pain that is difficult to control has become less common. However, in instances where it cannot be completely controlled, the risk of suicide often increases. In fact, a number of studies have found that most patients who committed suicide had inadequately controlled, severe pain (Massie, Gagnon, & Holland, 1994). Advanced cancer disease patients who have the highest suicide risk are more likely to have pain, depression, delirium, and various functional deficits (Crichton & Morley, 2002). Breitbart and Payne (1998) also noted that, besides pain, other factors associated with increased risk for suicide include the following: advanced illness and poor prognosis, depression and hopelessness, low sense of personal control and increased helplessness, low energy/exhaustion, a history of psychological disorders, past suicide attempts, and a family history of suicide.

Often, nursing and medical staff members are not adequately trained, or are inexperienced, in dealing with potential suicidal patients. A referral to a mental health specialist is therefore important if there is any suspicion of suicidal risk. Crichton and Morley (2002) provided two checklists of questions to use in a preliminary assessment of suicide risks:

1. A graded hierarchy of questions about current suicidal ideas and intent, such as "Have you ever felt in the last few days or weeks that you would just like to go to sleep and not wake up?" Follow-up questions would include "Do you think you might ever do anything to harm yourself?"
2. Questions about the factors discussed earlier that are associated with increased suicide risk (e.g., advanced illness and poor prognosis, depression and hopelessness, etc.) should then be asked.

If the risk for suicide is deemed high, then careful monitoring of the patient in the medical ward or at home by a mental health professional is essential. Often, antidepressant treatment may help, as might an increase in pain control and an opportunity for crisis-oriented therapy.

SUMMARY

Palliative care has now taken on a more substantial role for patients with pain, especially those with chronic, unremitting pain and cancer pain. Although palliative care does not necessarily cure the patient, or even extend the life of a patient, there is growing support for the premise that the quality of life for both the patient and his or her family can be significantly improved. This is actually a new orientation in medicine in general because, as people live longer, there is a growing development of chronic diseases that cannot be cured (e.g., hypertension, diabetes, asthma, arthritis), but merely managed. There is now a greater emphasis on developing more effective chronic disease management techniques, including that for palliative care of chronic pain.

REFERENCES

Abraham, J. L., & Snyder, L. (2001). Pain assessment and management. *Primary Care: Clinics in Office Practice, 28*, 17–38.

Adams, L. L., Gatchel, R. J., Robinson, R. C., Polatin, P. B., Gajraj, N., Deschner, M., et al. (2004). Development of a self-report screening instrument for assessing potential opioid medication misuse in chronic pain patients. *Journal of Pain and Symptom Management, 27*, 440–59.

American Society of Anesthesiologists Task Force on Pain Management. (1996). American Society of Anesthesiologists Task Force on Pain Management: Practice guidelines. *Anesthesiology, 84*, 1243–1257.

Bennett, G. J. (2000). Update on the neurophysiology of pain transmission and modularization: Focus on the NMDA receptor. *Journal of Pain and Symptom Management, 19*, S2–S6.

Block, A. R., Gatchel, R. J., Deardorff, W., & Guyer, R. D. (2003). *The psychology of spine surgery*. Washington, DC: American Psychological Association.

Breitbart, W., & Payne, D. K. (1998). Pain. In J. Holland (Ed.), *Psycho-Oncology* (pp. 450–467). New York: Oxford University Press.

Cameron, T., & Elliott, S. (2002). Spinal cord stimulation. *Practical Pain Management, 2*, 13–15.

Carney, M. T., & Meier, D. E. (2000). Palliative care and end-of-life issues. *Anesthesiology Clinics of North America, 18*, 183–206.

Chang, H. M. (1999). Cancer pain management. *Medical Clinics of North America, 83*, 711–736.

Cherny, N. I., & Catane, R. (1996). Palliative medicine and medical oncologists: Defining the purview of care. *Hematology/Oncology Clinics of North America, 10*, 1–20.

Crichton, P., & Morley, S. (2002). Treating pain in cancer patients. In D. C. Turk & R. J. Gatchel (Eds.), *Psychological approaches to pain management: A practitioner's handbook* (2nd ed., pp. 501–514). New York: Guilford Press.

Deschner, M., & Polatin, P. B. (2000). Interdisciplinary programs: Chronic pain management. In T. G. Mayer, R. J. Gatchel, & P. B. Polatin (Eds.), *Occupational musculoskeletal disorders: Function, outcomes and evidence* (pp. 629–637). Philadelphia: Lippincott, Williams & Wilkins.

Doleys, D. M. (2002). Preparing patients for implantable technologies. In D. C. Turk & R. J. Gatchel (Eds.), *Psychological approaches to pain management* (2nd ed., pp. 334–348). New York: Guilford Press.

Garvin, J. R. (1999). Anesthesiology and palliative care. *Anesthesiology Clinics of North America, 17*, 467–477.

Gatchel, R. J. (2001). A biopsychosocial overview of pre-treatment screening of patients with pain. *Clinical Journal of Pain, 17*, 192–199.

Grabow, T. S., Tella, P. K., & Raja, S. N. (2003). Spinal cord stimulation for complex regional pain syndrome: An evidence-based medicine review of the literature. *Clinical Journal of Pain, 19*, 371–383.

Graves, K. D. (2003). Social cognitive theory and cancer patients' quality of life: A meta-analysis of psychological intervention components. *Health Psychology, 22*, 210–219.

Harden, R. N. (2002). Chronic opioid therapy: Another reappraisal. *APS Bulletin, 12*, 1–12.

Hassenbusch, S. J., & Portenoy, R. K. (2000). Current practices and intraspinal therapy—Survey of clinical trials and decision making. *Journal of Pain and Symptom Management, 20*, S4–S11.

Hewitt, D. J. (2001). The management of pain in the oncology patient. *Obstetrics and Gynecology Clinics of North America, 28*, 314–323.

Joint Commission on Accreditation of Healthcare Organizations. (2000). *Pain assessment and management: An organizational approach*. Oakbrook, IL: Author.

Lipman, A. G. (2002). Pain management and palliative care: A natural—and needed—synergy. *APS Bulletin, 12,* 3–17.

Long, D. M. (1998). The current status of electrical stimulation of the nervous system for the relief of chronic pain. *Surgical Neurology, 49,* 142–144.

Massie, M., Gagnon, P., & Holland, J. (1994). Depression and suicide in patients with cancer. *Journal of Pain and Symptom Management, 9,* 325–331.

Melzack, R., & Wall, P. D. (1965). Pain mechanisms: A new theory. *Science, 50,* 971–979.

Nelson, D. V., Kennington, M., Novy, D. M., & Squitieri, P. (1996). Psychological selection criteria for implantable spinal cord stimulators. *Pain Forum, 5,* 93–103.

Noe, C. E., Gajraj, N. M., & Vakharia, A. S. (2000). Injection procedures. In T. G. Mayer, R. J. Gatchel, & P. B. Polatin (Eds.), *Occupational musculoskeletal disorders: Function, outcomes and evidence* (pp. 447–460). Philadelphia: Lippincott, Williams & Wilkins.

North, R. B., Kidd, D. H., Zahurak, M., James, C. S., & Long, D. M. (1993). Spinal cord stimulation for chronic, intractable pain: Experience over two decades. *Neurosurgery, 32,* 384–394.

Oliver, R. L., & Taylor, A. (2003, March/April). Chronic opioid rules. *Practical Pain Management,* 30–36.

Prager, J., & Jacobs, M. (2001). Evaluation of patients for implantable pain modalities: Medical and behavioral assessment. *Clinical Journal of Pain, 17,* 206–214.

Robinson, R. C., Gatchel, R. J., Polatin, P. B., Deschner, M., & Noe, C. (2001). Screening for problematic prescription opioid use. *Clinical Journal of Pain, 17,* 220–228.

Shealy, S., Mortimer, J. T., & Rewick, J. B. (1967). Electrical inhibition of pain by stimulation of the dorsal columns. *Anesthesia and Analgesia, 46,* 489–491.

Taylor, N. (1965). *Plant drugs that changed the world.* New York: Dodd, Mead, & Co.

Tennant, F., Liu, J., & Hermann, L. (2002). Intractable pain. *Practical Pain Management, 2,* 8–11.

World Health Organization Expert Committee. (1990). *Cancer pain relief and palliative care* (Technical Report Series 804). Geneva, Switzerland: World Health Organization.

Young, R. C., & Ades, T. B. (2001, September/October). Cancer pain: Successful management of patients' fears. *Practical Pain Management,* 8–13.

APPENDIX 9.1

Recommended Readings

Adams, L. L., Gatchel, R. J., Robinson, R. C., Polatin, P. B., Gajraj, N., Deschner, M., et al. (in press). Development of a self-report screening instrument for assessing potential opioid medication misuse in chronic pain patients. *Journal of Pain and Symptom Management*.

American Society of Anesthesiologists Task Force on Pain Management. (1996). American Society of Anesthesiologists Task Force on Pain Management: Practice guidelines. *Anesthesiology, 84,* 1243–1257.

Lipman, A. G. (2002). Pain management and palliative care: A natural—and needed—synergy. *APS Bulletin, 12,* 3–17.

Oliver, R. L., & Taylor, A. (2003, January/February). Chronic opioid rules. *Practical Pain Management,* 30–36.

10

REIMBURSEMENT ISSUES IN PAIN MANAGEMENT

Penny saved is a penny got.

—Henry Fielding, *The Miser*

Reimbursement issues are obviously extremely important for the viability of any pain management program or service. Currently, the declining reimbursement patterns and denial of treatment still remain the number-one problem for comprehensive pain management programs, with the average cost of care falling 32% since 1998 (Marketdata Enterprises, 2001). Overall, this cost has dropped by 5.7% per year since 1991. This has been due primarily to managed-care cost-containment pressures as well as to the entry of a greater number of anesthesiologists creating their own pain practices, which are usually less costly than multidisciplinary programs requiring larger staff sizes. Therefore, capturing every practice dollar is vital for the survival of a pain management program. In this chapter, I review issues such as appropriate Current Procedural Terminology (CPT) billing codes and different reimbursement strategies to use with various payers (i.e., Medicare, HMOs with and without carve-outs, workers' compensation systems, etc.). Most health care providers have never received any training in these billing/reimbursement issues and, therefore, are at a disadvantage with many third-party payers, who often take an adversarial role in denying treatment. This chapter is intended to provide important education concerning these matters. Varga (in press) also provided a good overview of issues associated with starting a pain management practice.

FINANCIAL STRUCTURE MODELS FOR PAIN MANAGEMENT SERVICES

Gatchel and Oordt (2003) provided an overview of the possible financial structure models that may be potentially used for primary-care psychology services. Such models can also be generalized for pain management services. These include the following and are discussed below:

- *Colocated clinics/centers model.* This model involves a pain management clinic or center that is colocated with a medical clinic or center or a hospital from which patients with pain may be referred. Of course, pain patients may be referred from a variety of other sources as well. The pain management and medical clinics may share appointment and reception services and waiting rooms, but they remain two separate organizations. This colocation alone may also provide several other advantages. Referrals between clinics and centers may be easier, especially if one scheduling system is used. The medical and pain management providers will become familiar with one another's work, and communication between the two is likely to be facilitated by physical colocation. This frequently improves collaboration and enhances the patient's perception that all aspects of health care are being well coordinated.
- *Pain management and the primary-provider model.* This model entails the pain management clinic or center as a stand-alone facility. Patients are referred from various outside sources, and they receive all their comprehensive assessment and treatment at this clinic or center. This is the usual model of interdisciplinary pain management centers.
- *Pain management consultant model.* This model involves a pain management specialist as a consultant who may be called on by various health care professionals and facilities to provide expertise for pain management, when needed, in the overall health care plan for certain patients. The consultant sees patients for evaluation and makes recommendations to the referring health care professional, who then becomes responsible for providing and coordinating the recommended care. The consultant may follow the patient to monitor, or even help in the implementation of, the recommendations. In seeing patients for follow-up, the consultant may collaborate in providing pain management interventions while maintaining communication about the patient's progress and treatment plan with the physician, who remains the primary decision maker.
- *Combination of models.*

All of the models discussed above are not necessarily mutually exclusive. Each offers the opportunity for providing assessment and treatment services for patients with pain. A stepped-care approach may be used. For example, a pain treatment center may request a consultant to provide assessment services and then provide a treatment plan. If it is subsequently found that the patient does not make the desired changes, the consultant may be requested to interview the patient again to further assess the problem and refine the intervention. If again there is not sufficient improvement, the center may decide to bring the consultant in to actually engage the patient in the treatment protocol.

Financial Issues

The specific model chosen may depend largely on financial issues related to different types of practice, because different systems of health care will support integrated health care professionals differently. Some practices are based on *fee for service*. In these settings, providers bill patients or insurance companies for the services provided. One disadvantage of this is that these individual services often have to be preauthorized and precertified for every single session. Moreover, third-party payers typically exclude certain services from reimbursement. For example, Medicare specifically excludes "consultation" services and psychophysiological therapy (e.g., biofeedback training for headaches or anxiety), as well as the majority of preventive services and across-the-board screenings (American Psychological Association Practice Directorate, 2001). Furthermore, in the past few years, many insurance plans have changed their policies so they now only reimburse psychologists for *mental health care* (using psychiatric codes). As a result, psychologists who want to work with traditional medical disorders, such as pain, have encountered more difficulty with third-party payment. Psychologists working in a fee-for-service practice have sometimes had to limit their practice to treatment of primary or comorbid mental health disorders (e.g., treating major depression in patients with chronic pain, or adjustment disorders in newly diagnosed patients with pain) in order to get reimbursed (Gatchel & Oordt, 2003). Fortunately, in January 2002, six new CPT codes became available for assessment and interventions with physical health patients (see Table 10.1). Nonphysician health care professionals, who are intimately involved in pain management programs (e.g., psychologists, nurses, social workers, and physical therapists) need to be aware of these new CPT codes under which they can bill. This will allow them to bill for services directed at physical health issues such as pain, and it eliminates the need for a mental health diagnosis for psychological services to be reimbursed (Smith, 2002). However, keep in mind that the *rate* of reimbursement is still at issue. Medicare may have mandated its fee schedules, but

TABLE 10.1
Current Procedural Terminal Terminology (CPT) Codes Available for Behavioral, Social, and Psychophysiological Assessment and Interventions for the Prevention, Treatment, and Management of Physical Health Problems

CPT code	Service provided	Approximate Medicare payment per 15-min unit
96150	Assessment, initial	$26
96151	Reassessment	$26
96152	Intervention, individual	$25
96153	Intervention, group (per person)	$5
96154	Intervention, family with patient	$24
96155	Intervention, family without patient	$23

many major private insurers may not have yet done so. Therefore, it behooves each health care professional to practice due diligence by checking with each insurance payer as to whether it reimburses these codes and, if so, at what rate. A decision regarding the practicality of using these rates at this point in time can then be made on a case-by-case (or insurance carrier-by-carrier) basis.

Unfortunately, the psychological codes are reimbursed at significantly lower levels than would be paid if nonphysician pain specialists were reimbursed for using medical CPT codes. Despite the fact that payers have begun refusing payment on claims in which psychologists, for example, have used medical codes, psychologists specializing in pain management should continue to advocate for reimbursement on these higher paying codes. Facts that justify the use of these codes by psychologists, suggested by W. Deardorff (personal communication, January 2002), include the following:

- Within the scope of their license, psychologists can provide treatment for physical problems. This treatment is not psychotherapy, and it does not address mental health problems (of course, when the nature of treatment is psychotherapy, it is then more appropriate to bill it as such). Laws are now in effect in most states that prohibit discrimination of reimbursement based on the degree the provider holds (e.g., PhD vs. MD), as long as the treatment provided is within the scope of the provider's training and expertise.
- It is not necessarily fair to patients to bill using a psychiatric diagnosis and treatment code if this is not the situation. Many patients would prefer not to have a psychiatric diagnosis in their medical charts that might "follow them" during subsequent years.

- In light of what is known about the benefits and cost-effectiveness of many pain assessment and management services provided by psychologists, a payer's unwillingness to reimburse psychologists for these services represents a lack of commitment to quality, cost-effective care. It also reflects an unjust two-tiered system in which insurers are more reluctant to reimburse psychological services than medical services. Total allowable charges for psychological services are significantly less than for medical services with most insurance plans.

Appendix 10.2 contains the primary psychological codes that my colleagues and I are currently using at our pain management center.

Medicare Issues

It is also important to know that when providing care to Medicare beneficiaries, such services for those patients will be reimbursed at a higher rate than the psychotherapy code because, under current federal regulations, an outpatient mental health treatment limitation does not apply to these new services (American Psychological Association, 2002). It applies only to those services provided to patients with a mental, psychoneurotic, or personality disorder (identified by an ICD-9 CM diagnosis code between 290 and 319). As an example, Medicare will reduce the approved amount of a 45-min outpatient psychotherapy session by 62.5% and then reimburse 80% of the remainder (resulting in a final payment of approximately $48). In contrast, Medicare will reimburse a 45-min outpatient health and behavior intervention session for an individual at 80% of the approved amount (approximately $59). As the American Psychological Association (2002) noted:

> Federal reimbursement for the health and behavior assessment and intervention codes will come out of funding for medical rather than psychiatric services and will not draw from limited mental health dollars. For private third-party insurance, we expect these services to be treated under the physical-illness benefits of a plan and thus not be subject to the higher outpatient consumer co-payment found in Medicare or relegated to the behavioral health "carve-out" provisions.

Independent Practice Versus Group Practice

Finally, it should be pointed out that nonphysician pain specialists, such as psychologists, who are attempting to integrate their practices into multidisciplinary private group practices may have an advantage over individuals in independent practice in terms of contracting with third-party payers. Some health-management companies, in forming their provider networks, may be more willing to contract with a relatively small number of group practices than with a large number of individual providers, thus making the integrated practice more attractive (American Psychological Association Practice Directorate, 2001). Laws differ in each state regarding how psychologists and physicians can associate in practice (i.e., partnerships, professional corporations, limited liability companies, etc.). Psychologists interested in these arrangements are referred to the publication *Models of Multidisciplinary Arrangements: A State-by-State Review of Options* (American Psychological Association Practice Directorate, 2001) and should also seek legal counsel.

Of course, psychologists must also attend to ethical concerns related to the financial aspects of practice. For example, psychologists must avoid splitting fees with physicians or other health care providers with whom they work collaboratively or from whom they receive referrals. They also must not provide financial kickbacks to providers who refer patients for evaluation or treatment.

MARKETING AND PUBLIC RELATIONS TOOLS TO IMPROVE ONE'S PRACTICE

Of course, most practitioners would agree that building a responsive and successful pain management practice requires the ethical use of effective marketing, public relations, and advertising. As I discuss in the next chapter, the best advertisement is the availability of evidence-based successful outcome data that you can send to referral sources and to insurance payers. Wauford (in press) reviewed how to market pain management programs, and Rapp (2003) summarized a number of methods for marketing one's practice:

- *Develop a positive image.* Be certain that your receptionist or office operation is helpful and pleasant. Also be aware to make your telephone voicemail system user friendly.
- *Develop a Web site for your practice.* In doing so, be certain that you respond quickly to information requests made via the Web site.
- *Host open houses for both insurance providers and referral sources.* During these open houses, have information available about your program, its success, and your referral feedback process. Also, it is often helpful to develop a "patient of the month" program and invite such patients to the open house.

- *Participate in local health care and pain support group events.* Attending such events regularly is a good way to "get your name out there." Also, regularly attend local and state meetings of professional organizations where pain management is represented.
- *Be media savvy.* Try to develop good relations with the local media. This might mean offering to write articles for newspapers or making yourself available if information about pain is needed. If possible, bring local media representatives together for an open house to update their knowledge of what you are doing.
- *Develop a newsletter for your practice* in which you discuss any new developments, procedures offered, and so on. Also include patient success stories as well as any new outcome data demonstrating the success of your program. Send it to former patients (who are often useful in referring friends); your current referral sources; potential referral sources; and insurance company case managers, who are often gatekeepers.

THE PROBLEM OF CARVE-OUTS

One major obstacle pain management specialists will encounter is that insurance companies often contract the management of specific services, such as mental and behavioral services, to a separate mental health management company, often referred to as a mental health *carve-out*. This can also be true for physical therapy and occupational therapy services. Patients maintain maximum benefit by using a professional who is on the panel of the preferred-provider network rather than paying higher out-of-pocket costs for an out-of-network professional. For most pain specialists, it is therefore quite important to get on as many of these provider panels as possible.

Keep in mind that psychologists will need to verify coverage and obtain preauthorization *and* precertification before seeing patients, both to ensure benefits for their patients as well as to protect themselves financially (simply receiving preauthorization does not guarantee payment for services; precertification is ultimately needed). Unfortunately, this may prevent patients from being seen on a same-day basis. The patient's insurance card typically has the contact information if a different company manages mental and behavioral services, physical therapy services, and so on. Another caveat is that *preauthorization* is a term usually used only with workers' compensation carriers, and it reflects a commitment by the carrier to pay for specific services requested by the health care provider. However, it is *not* a full guarantee of payment (many carriers may fall back on the phrase "reasonable and necessary" services; however, this is a fairly rare occurrence). *Precertification* has come to be used in much the same way as *preauthorization*, although carriers are really "preauthorizing" a specified number of sessions (thereby indicating their commitment to pay for the services after they have been rendered). Some carriers, though, still use *precertification* in its original sense (i.e., to certify that a given patient has benefits with that company). By using the term in this way, they are making no commitment ahead of time to pay for specific services the health care professional wishes to provide. It is incumbent on the health care professional and his or her billing staff to be aware of the different nuances in how these terms are used and how they may vary from one insurance carrier to the next. This homework is essential for the financial survival of a practice or clinic.

Recent research has demonstrated that carve-out policies can significantly compromise the effectiveness of pain management programs (Gatchel et al., 2001; Robbins et al., 2003). For example, Robbins et al. (2003) found that physical therapy carve-out practices had a negative impact on both the short-term and 1-year follow-up outcome measures in patients undergoing an interdisciplinary pain management program. Thus, such insurance carrier policies of contracting treatment carve-outs significantly compromise the efficacy of an evidence-based, best-standard medical care treatment such as interdisciplinary care for pain. This raises important medico–legal and ethical issues, as well as vocational implications, for patients' long-term improvement and independent financial security. This attempt to contain costs in the short term is also shortsighted, because chronic pain will continue to be a medical problem requiring additional future long-term treatment costs. With the new "Pain Care Bill of Rights" issued by the American Pain Foundation, chronic-pain patients are now in a position to begin demanding the best standard of care for their chronic pain (i.e., interdisciplinary pain management). Other clinical researchers have also demonstrated the negative impact on outcomes by not providing full integrated interdisciplinary care for pain patients when it is required (e.g., Keel et al., 1998).

Another strategy to avoid carve-out policies is to get on insurance panels as a provider of a specific service (i.e., interdisciplinary pain management) instead of a piecemeal program (with separate medical, psychological, physical therapy, and occupational therapy services). Many times, it is a matter of strongly negotiating contracts with insurance carriers to get this type of specific bundling of services as part of their panels. However, it is important to never sign a managed-care contract without careful scrutiny of the services that can be provided as well as provider compensation. Managed-care organization contracts may often be quite deceptive in these areas (Montgomery, 2002).

There are major problems for coordinated care when insurance "carve-outs" are imposed on patients.

REIMBURSEMENT ISSUES IN OTHER MODELS OF CARE

Staff-model systems are likely to provide more options for nonphysician pain specialists than preferred-provider networks (Gatchel & Oordt, 2003; Strosahl, 1998). A staff-model system is one in which providers are salaried by a health care organization that is responsible for the total health care of a specified population of patients. Examples of these include HMOs, such as Kaiser Permanente and Group Health Cooperative, and federal systems such as the Veterans Administration and the military health care systems. Indeed, integrated care was originally spawned in this type of system and has blossomed within several of them. The financial structure of these systems reinforces health care initiatives that help maintain optimal health in their populations and minimize the occurrence of chronic and severe disease that often results in costly care. Fortunately, preliminary data are available to support the potential for health care organizations to save money in the long run (i.e., cost offset) by effectively meeting the psychosocial needs of patients (Gatchel & Oordt, 2003). Reviews of this literature have been presented by Strosahl (1998), who concluded that such integrated care can achieve medical cost offsets and also improve the quality of care delivered by providers.

UNDERSTANDING THE MEDICO–LEGAL SYSTEM

Before leaving this issue of reimbursement policies, it is important to fully understand the medico–legal system that has jurisdiction over the patient's case. The jurisdictions that are most commonly encountered in the United States (and those subject to the system), as delineated by Leeman, Polatin, Gatchel, and Kishino (2000), are listed in Exhibit 10.1. Quite often, the specific treatment benefits that are allowed under each system may or may not be fully understood by patients, who might need some education about what they can reasonably expect when their claims are resolved. Just as important is that each of the medico–legal jurisdictions is a distinct entity unto itself, with different service sectors, eligibility requirements, rules of engagement, and options for case resolution. Exhibit 10.1 also summarizes the major differences in these various systems. In addition, it should also be remembered that each state has its own workers' compensation system guidelines; there is no one general workers' compensation system covering all states.

PROPER CODING AND BILLING COMPLIANCE

Today, if one is involved in the delivery of any health care in the United States, then one automatically needs to be aware of the importance of coding. There has never been such an emphasis on the description and definition of what health care providers do for, and to, the patient as there is today. Correct coding is a necessity in today's health care system. Correct coding accompanying any billing for health care service is now a *legal requirement*. This legal requirement was instigated by governmental policy

EXHIBIT 10.1
Summary of Medico–Legal Jurisdictions

- *State Workers' Compensation.* Statutes governing benefits vary greatly from state to state.
- *Federal Employees Compensation Act.* Governs workers' compensation for federal employees, including postal workers and Veterans' Administration employees.
- *Federal Employees Labor Act.* Under this law, a claimant can pursue a "buyout," which typically results in litigation focusing on issues of disability and employability.
- *U.S. Longshore and Harbor Workers' Compensation Act and Jones Act.* Workers covered under these acts include those working offshore, in port, or aboard a ship; claimants may pursue large monetary settlements based on employability and disability factors.
- *Nonsubscriber and Personal Injury Litigation.* In those few states where workers' compensation is not mandatory (e.g., Texas), or for those injuries that fall outside the workers' compensation system, injured workers may seek a legal remedy through personal injury litigation. Disability, employability, lost wages, earning capacity, and pain and suffering are all relevant issues.
- *Short- and Long-Term Disability.* Such policies may provide financial support through age 65, provided the injured worker proves an inability to engage in his or her own occupation, depending on the terms of the particular policy.
- *Social Security Disability Insurance.* Provides federal disability retirement benefits on a monthly basis to individuals who are unable to work because of a disability.

Note. From "Managing Secondary Gain in Patients With Pain-Associated Disability: A Clinical Perspective," by G. Leeman, P. Polatin, R. Gatchel, and N. Kishino, Summer 2000, *Journal of Workers Compensation, 9,* pp. 25–44. Copyright 2000 by Standard Publishing Corp., Boston, MA. Adapted with permission.

in the form of two major acts/bills: (a) the Budget Reconciliation Act of 1997 and (b) the Kennedy–Kassebaum Health Reform Bill. The former empowered and directed the Centers for Medicare and Medicaid Services to develop a payment system based on documented health care professional work. The latter empowered and directed the Office of the Inspector General and the Federal Bureau of Investigation to identify and prosecute health care fraud and abuse. These two actions have established the requirement for the correct coding of assessment and treatment procedures. In light of the current climate in the health care field, it is essential for all types of practices to have an internal compliance plan, in addition to an active compliance program, to ensure that the practice is compliant with all of the federally mandated health care fraud and abuse laws. One such model— "Guidance for Individual and Small Group Physician Practices"—was produced by the Office of the Inspector General's draft of a model compliance program (for information, contact the American Medical Association, Customer Service, at 1-800-621-8335). This document outlines the specific components of a model compliance program plan.

With the significant legal ramifications, it is now just as important to have the billing staff of one's practice to be well trained in the appropriate coding terminology in order to provide a double check on the health care professional's coding and billing notes. This will provide a safeguard to ensure that appropriate codes and billing statements are consistently documented. Unannounced external audits are now quite frequent in health care facilities. Thus, a practitioner must be extremely diligent in making certain that the coding and billing guidelines are carefully adhered to. There are now a number of publications available that provide comprehensive pain management coding and billing rules for both Medicare and private payers, such as the *Pain Management Coding and Billing Answer Book* (National Pain Management Reimbursement Division, 2003).

Finally, besides the legal requirement of using proper coding and billing guidelines, health care professionals are also required to establish a minimum level of privacy protection for health care information of patients. The U.S. Department of Health and Human Services has developed the Health Insurance Portability and Accountability Act (HIPAA) Privacy Rule, which establishes patients' rights concerning the use and disclosure of their health care information. Access to patient data must be carefully controlled by health care providers, health care plans, and health care clearinghouses. The American Psychological Association has made information about HIPAA compliance available at the Web site http://www.apapractice.org. The actual HIPAA security rule issued by the Department of Health and Human Services was published in the *Federal Register* on February 20, 2003. Appendix 10.3 provides a summary of what a health care professional should do to be certain that he or she is compliant with HIPAA. An overview of the various legal, regulatory, and ethical issues associated with pain treatment programs discussed throughout this volume can also be found in Dunn (2003).

SUMMARY

In the current managed-care environment, to provide comprehensive pain management services is frequently problematic because of constraints on the initiation of a referral, authorization of appropriate treatment services, and reimbursement issues. Also, one needs to be aware of a number of legal, regulatory, and ethical issues relating to pain management (Dunn, 2003). Because pain is both a physical and psychological constellation of illness states, treatment needs to address both the *psyche* and the *soma,* using a biopsychosocial perspective. However, health care reimbursement frequently insists on a focus on one versus the other, forcing the clinician to go through an arduous process of justification and negotiation, sometimes to the extreme of altering one's pure biopsychosocial perspective in the service of obtaining good patient care. This state of affairs often reflects a lack of basic understanding on the part of the insurance adjusters, who are unschooled in the subtleties of pain management or who may not be open to such education.

In fact, pain management may be considered a low priority, particularly in the private sector, where there is no appeal process for a denial of care. In other venues of health care, such as workers' compensation, the Veterans' Administration, and the Department of Labor, there is an appeal process, which must be followed in the interest of being a true patient advocate.

It is, therefore, important that clinicians who are attempting to provide pain management services be aware of the obstacles of the medical marketplace and be able to negotiate without becoming frustrated or angry, in a good-faith effort to provide treatment, educate the lay community, and inform patients of obstacles interfering with comprehensive treatment. If one has exhausted all of one's resources with good documentation of one's efforts, then it may be necessary to shift the burden to a motivated patient to continue the lobbying efforts on his or her own behalf. The ultimate goal is to get treatment authorized and then to get it reimbursed. Finally, it cannot be overemphasized that it is extremely important for health care professionals to exert great effort to become very knowledgeable about whatever insurance system(s) they choose to bill under. This initial drudgery of learning the system(s) ultimately pays off later in increased collection rates.

REFERENCES

American Medical Association. (2003). *Current procedural terminology: CPT 2003, standard edition.* Chicago: Author.

American Psychological Association. (2002). APA Practice Directorate announces new health and behavior CPT codes. *PsychNET.* Retrieved April 21, 2004, from http://www.apa.org/practice/cpt—2002.html

American Psychological Association Practice Directorate. (2001). *Models for multidisciplinary arrangements: A state-by-state review of opinions.* Washington, DC: Author.

Dunn, P. M. (2003). Legal landscape of pain treatment. *Practical Pain Management, 3,* 12–17.

Gatchel, R. J., Noe, C., Gajraj, N. M., Vakharia, A. S., Polatin, P. B., Deschner, M., et al. (2001). Treatment carve-out practices: Their effect on managing pain at an interdisciplinary pain center. *Journal of Workers Compensation, 10,* 50–63.

Gatchel, R. J., & Oordt, M. S. (2003). *Clinical health psychology and primary care: Practical advice and clinical guidance for successful collaboration.* Washington, DC: American Psychological Association.

Health Insurance Portability and Accountability Act of 1996—Security Standards, 68 Fed. Reg. 34, 8333-8399 (Feb. 20, 2003).

Keel, P., Wittig, R., Deutschman, R., Diethelm, U., Knusel, O., Loschmann, C., et al. (1998). Effectiveness of in-patient rehabilitation for sub-chronic and chronic low back pain by an integrative group treatment program. *Scandinavian Journal of Rehabilitation Medicine, 30,* 211–219.

Leeman, G., Polatin, P., Gatchel, R., & Kishino, N. (2000). Managing secondary gain in patients with pain-associated disability: A clinical perspective. *Journal of Workers Compensation, 9,* 25–44.

Marketdata Enterprises. (2001). *Chronic pain management clinics: A market analysis.* Tampa, FL: Author.

Montgomery, S. P. (2002, November/December). Managed care contract review. *Spineline, 33–34.*

National Pain Management Reimbursement Division. (2003). *Pain management coding and billing answer book.* Gaithersburg, MD: Author.

Rapp, S. M. (2003, August). Marketing, PR, advertising tools available to build any practice. *Orthopedics Today, 30.*

Robbins, H., Gatchel, R. J., Noe, C., Gajraj, N., Polatin, P., Deschner, M., et al. (2003). A prospective one-year outcome study of interdisciplinary chronic pain management: Compromising its efficacy by managed care policies. *Anesthesia & Analgesia, 97,* 156–162.

Smith, D. (2002, May). Lessons learned from Sept. 11: Psychologists' research uncovers our strengths and weaknesses. *Monitor on Psychology, 34–35.*

Strosahl, K. (1998). Integrating behavioral health and primary care services: The primary mental health care model. In A. Blount (Ed.), *Integrated primary care: The future of medical and mental health collaboration* (pp. 139–166). New York: W. W. Norton.

Varga, C. (in press). Starting a pain clinic. In B. E. Cole & M. Boswell (Eds.), *Pain management: A practical guide for clinicians* (7th ed.). Boca Raton, FL: CRC Press.

Wauford, K. (in press). Marketing pain management programs. In B. E. Cole & M. Boswell (Eds.), *Pain management: A practical guide for clinicians* (7th ed.). Boca Raton, FL: CRC Press.

APPENDIX 10.1

Recommended Readings

American Psychological Association Practice Directorate. (2001). *Models for multi-disciplinary arrangements: A state-by-state review of options.* Washington, DC: Author.

Dunn, P. M. (2003). Legal landscape of pain treatment. *Practical Pain Management, 3,* 12–17.

Gatchel, R. J., & Oordt, M. S. (2003). *Clinical health psychology and primary care: Practical advice and clinical guidance for successful collaboration.* Washington, DC: American Psychological Association.

National Pain Management Reimbursement Division. (2003). *Pain management coding and billing answer book.* Gaithersburg, MD: Author.

Robbins, H., Gatchel, R. J., Noe, C., Gajraj, N., Polatin, P., Deschner, M., et al. (2003). A prospective one-year outcome study of interdisciplinary chronic pain management: Compromising its efficacy by managed care policies. *Anesthesia & Analgesia, 97,* 156–162.

Wauford, K. (in press). Marketing pain management programs. In B. E. Cole & M. Boswell (Eds.), *Pain management: A practical guide for clinicians* (7th ed.). Boca Raton, FL: CRC Press.

APPENDIX 10.2

Primary Psychological Codes

Evaluation Codes

The following two codes (90801 & 96100) constitute the **Behavioral Medicine Evaluation,** described as the following (90801, 96100 × 2 hours):

Description

A one-time-only, psychiatric diagnostic interview, personality testing (MMPI–2 and MBMD), depression rating scales, and pain and disability coping scales.

Purpose

Provide the referring party with a comprehensive evaluation of psychological factors that are influencing response to injury and/or illness and affecting the patient's recovery. Interview includes history of injury/illness and present symptoms, the effect on physical and mental functioning, current activities and limitations, personal and family psychiatric history, substance abuse history, psychosocial history, and mental status. In the case of workers' compensation, a determination of the relationship of current psychological status to injury- and noninjury-related factors is also made. The focus of the evaluation is to provide the referring physician with practical treatment recommendations for speeding recovery, including psychological, behavioral pain management, general rehabilitation, and patient management issues. Reports are generally 4–6 pages.

Diagnostic Interview (CPT–90801) × 90 minutes

- "Psychiatric diagnostic interview examination includes a history, mental status, and a disposition, and may include communication with family or other sources, ordering and medical interpretation of laboratory or other medical diagnostic studies" (American Medical Association, 2003, p. 292).

Psychological Testing With Report (CPT–96100) × 2 hours

- "Psychological testing (includes psychodiagnostic assessment of personality, psychopathology, emotionality, intellectual abilities, e.g., WAIS–R, Rorschach, MMPI) *with interpretation and report, per hour*" (American Medical Association, 2003, p. 317).
  - *This charge entails face-to-face work with the client, plus the time the clinician spends interpreting and writing up the report of test findings. This means that the clinician needs to be able to prove that the bulk of the two-hour charge was spent interpreting the data and writing the report, as we do not conduct face-to-face testing evaluations, e.g. as in intelligence testing.*

Therapy Codes

Individual Psychotherapy (CPT–90806) × _____ 45–50 minute sessions

Individual Psychotherapy (CPT–90804) × _____ 20–30 minute sessions

- "Individual psychotherapy, insight oriented, behavior modifying and/or supportive, in an office or outpatient facility, approximately 45–50 (or 20–30 minutes, using code 90804) minutes face-to face with the patient" (American Medical Association, 2003, p. 293).

Description

Consists of psychotherapy sessions utilizing a cognitive–behavioral approach to reduce depression, anxiety, fear, etc., that stems from the injury/illness and/or is impeding the patient's ability to derive maximum benefit from rehabilitation efforts or are hindering return to work. Where appropriate, behavioral pain management techniques are also included (muscle relaxation training, breathing, and imagery). The focus of therapy is on removing barriers to recovery and return to productive lifestyle, as well as a return to pre-injury psychological functioning. Patients are usually seen once a week. Clinical documentation of the patient's attendance, progress, and need for further treatment will be maintained. Length of treatment varies with patients' status, but is reassessed regularly.

Note. MMPI–2 = Minnesota Multiphasic Personality Inventory—2; MBMD = Millon Behavioral Medical Diagnostic; WAIS–R = Wechsler Adult Intelligence Scale—Revised.

APPENDIX 10.3

Summary of Ways to Become HIPAA Compliant

- Post your "Notice of Privacy Practices" in a clear, prominent location.
- Give patients copies of your "Notice of Privacy Practices," and make good-faith efforts to obtain written evidence of their receipt.
- Avoid verbal discussions of protected health information (PHI) on the phone or in reception/waiting areas that are within earshot of people who do not have a need to know.
- Do not leave PHI on telephone answering machines.
- Do not include PHI announcements made in your waiting rooms.
- Try to get some sense of whether your patients want you discussing their PHI with their family and friends, and restrict information if not.
- Limit (or, to the extent possible, eliminate) patient information on whiteboards, x-ray boxes, computer screens, and other areas that may be visible to the public and others who do not need access to PHI.
- Follow safeguards for PHI that is transmitted by fax or e-mail (or prohibit these activities until prudent safeguards can be put in place).
- File away promptly (and lock at night) folders that contain patient medical records.
- Make sure the physical plant is locked down at night, with windows closed and doors locked.
- Remove signage that would help an ill-intentioned person to find PHI (e.g., a sign on the patients' records department that reads "Confidential Patient Information").

- Remind people that only the minimum necessary PHI should be disclosed to anyone.
- Make sure all workforce members who leave your employment turn in their keys and building cards and lose their network connection privileges.
- Make sure written authorizations to use and disclose PHI are received for treatment, payment, operations, and exceptions.
- Make sure new and existing employees are aware of your schedule for ongoing HIPAA privacy training.
- Make sure everyone is aware of the rights patients have to review (and get copies of) their records and what procedures will be followed.
- Make sure everyone knows with whom patients should speak if they have questions about their HIPAA privacy rights.
- Be sure everyone in your workforce knows who your privacy officer is and whom they should contact with patient privacy questions or problems or if someone has a complaint or wants to report a violation of your organization's privacy policies or procedures.

IV

THE FUTURE OF PAIN MANAGEMENT

11

FUTURE NEEDS AND DIRECTIONS OF PAIN MANAGEMENT

Knowledge is experience. . . . Everything else is just information.
—Albert Einstein

The essence of knowledge is, having it, to apply it; not having it, to confess your ignorance.
—Confucius

As I have reviewed elsewhere (Gatchel, 1999), and discussed in chapter 1, many historical changes have occurred in medicine in general, including pain medicine, during the past centuries. During the Renaissance, the perspective that the mind (or the soul) influenced the body was regarded as unscientific. The goal of understanding the mind and soul was viewed as the purview of religion and philosophy; the understanding of the body was viewed as a separate realm of the growing field of physical medicine. This was a result of the new approach to the investigation of physical phenomena that emerged during this period. This viewpoint initiated the trend toward a *biomedical reductionism* approach, which argued that concepts such as the mind and the soul were not needed to explain physical functioning or behavior. Unfortunately, this new mechanistic approach to the study of human anatomy and physiology also fostered a dualistic viewpoint that the mind and body function separately and independently.

The influence of this strict mechanistic, dualistic approach to medicine began to subside during the late 19th and early 20th centuries. Influential writings began to appear that emphasized the importance of taking an integrated, more holistic approach to health and illness. A more comprehensive *biopsychosocial model* of illness was proposed that emphasized the unique interaction of biological, physiological, and psychosocial factors that need to be taken into account for a better understanding of health and illness.

Of course, conventional medicine has always been slow to change, and it is only now that this biopsychosocial perspective is gaining greater acceptance in the medical community. One of the reasons for this increasing acceptance of such a biopsychosocial perspective has been the increasing prevalence of chronic medical disorders in the United States. Indeed, with the increase in size of the aging population in this country, the prevalence of chronic medical conditions can be expected to continue to rise. As of 2001, approximately 35 million Americans, age 65 years or older, accounted for 12.4% of the total population (U.S. Census Bureau, 2001). It has been projected that by the year 2030 approximately 20% of the population will be 65 years or older (U.S. Census Bureau, 2000). Awareness of these population trends is contributing to increased concern about health care for older adults, because these older individuals are likely to have a high prevalence of chronic medical problems, such as chronic pain. Also, as I have discussed throughout this book, pain conditions require a comprehensive biopsychosocial approach to assessment and treatment. Moreover, chronic pain conditions usually cannot be *cured*; instead, they can be merely *treated* or *managed*.

Although the area of pain management has evidenced significant advances during the past decade, there are some important issues and topics that require additional attention because of their important clinical relevance. I discuss these next.

MATCHING THE RIGHT TREATMENT WITH THE RIGHT PATIENT

As I have discussed throughout this book, there is no question that psychosocial and behavioral factors play a significant role in the perception of, experience of, and response to pain. Research has revealed that groups of patients may differ in psychosocial and behavioral characteristics, even when the medical diagnosis is identical (e.g., Turk & Gatchel, 1999b). Likewise, individuals with the same medical diagnosis may vary greatly in their response to their symptoms. Turk and his colleagues, for example, have revealed that patients with diseases and syndromes as varied as back pain, headache, and metastatic cancer may display comparable adaptation patterns, whereas patients with the same diagnosis may actually show great variability in their degree of disability (e.g., Turk & Gatchel, 1999b; Turk, Okifuji, Sinclair, & Starz, 1998).

As Turk and Gatchel (1999b) indicated, the traditional approach of lumping together patients with the same medical diagnosis or set of symptoms (e.g., back pain, fibromyalgia, temporomandibular disorder), and then to treat them all the same way, is not appropriate, because many of these common diagnoses are relatively gross categories, and there may be unique individual differences of patients who fall under these generic diagnoses. Thus, some patients may respond quite positively to a certain treatment, whereas others may actually show no improvement at all. Therefore, it is becoming more important to match a particular intervention to specific patient characteristics. As Turk (1990) originally emphasized, the myth of "pain patient homogeneity" must be debunked, and patient differences need to be taken into account in order to tailor an appropriate treatment program. Turk and Okifuji (2001) provided a comprehensive review of the importance of the treatment-matching process and literature to support greater clinical efficacy of such a matching-approach strategy.

A number of studies have already demonstrated that patients classified into different subgroups based on their behavioral and psychosocial characteristics respond differentially to identical treatments (Epker & Gatchel, 2000; Turk, 2002). This has been fairly consistently observed across different types of pain syndromes (e.g., cancer, fibromyalgia, headache, low back pain, and temporomandibular joint pain). The differences in the psychosocial profiles displayed by patients has led to attempts to categorize different subgroups of patients and then to evaluate differential response to a treatment. For example, as I reviewed in chapter 4, several outcome studies have demonstrated the effective use of the Multidimensional Pain Inventory (MPI; Kerns, Turk, & Rudy, 1985) as one way to categorize subgroups of patients. Turk and Okifuji (1998) reviewed additional research demonstrating the utility of the MPI with other chronic pain conditions, including headache, temporomandibular joint pain, and fibromyalgia. Assessment of such MPI profiles will help tailor the needs for treatment strategies to account for the different personality characteristics of patients. For example, patients with an interpersonally distressed profile may need additional clinical attention addressing interpersonal skills to perform effectively in a group-oriented treatment program. Pain patients with dysfunctional and interpersonally distressed profiles display more indications of acute and chronic personality differences, relative to adaptive-coper profile patients, and they therefore require more clinical management (e.g., Etscheidt, Steiger, & Braverman, 1995). Such additional attention, however, would not necessarily be essential for adaptive-coper profile patients.

Studies such as the ones just discussed support the notion that, because patients' responses to treatment differ as a function of their psychosocial coping profiles, then specific treatment modalities are more likely than others to be better suited to each profile. An important issue for future clinical research is whether there are other types of biopsychosocial profiles that are more or less responsive to different treatment modalities. For example, variables that have been found to be predictors of pain-related disability outcomes, such as catastrophizing, fear of movement/reinjury, pain beliefs, anxiety and depression, and so on, and their interactions with environmental factors, such as workplace variables, health care system variables, and so on, need to be more closely evaluated (Turk & Monarch, 2002).

Finally, one additional important area of treatment matching involves the patient's readiness to accept a self-management pain approach, which may be conceptualized in terms of Prochaska and DiClemente's (1983) *transtheoretical model of stages of change*, discussed in chapter 7. Kerns, Rosenberg, Jamison, Caudill, and Haythornthwaite (1997) proposed that these readiness-to-change stages are important in deciding what treatment strategies need to be applied to particular patients. For example, patients in the *precontemplation stage* may embrace a belief that the pain problem is purely a medical one and that medical professionals are expected to treat and cure it. The learning of pain self-management skills may be viewed as useless and, therefore, beginning this type of treatment will probably lead to noncompliance and failure. In contrast, patients in the *action stage* are more likely to accept the need for a self-management approach, and they will conscientiously engage in efforts to acquire new coping skills and embrace the program as a whole. Finally, patients in the *maintenance stage* are likely to have a genuine belief in the effectiveness of self-management and will simply need guidance in continuing to consolidate and expand their skills. Thus, tailoring the treatment to the patient's stage of readiness to change will allow a more efficient and time-effective tailoring of pain management program components to that patient. The Pain Stages of Change Questionnaire was developed for this purpose (Kerns et al., 1997).

THE IMPORTANCE OF TREATMENT OUTCOMES EVALUATION

As Mayer, Gatchel, and Polatin (2000) noted, health care costs are continuing to increase at an alarming rate in the United States. Therefore, changes in health care policy and demands for improved allocations of health resources have recently placed great pressure on health care professionals to provide the most cost-effective treatment for pain syndromes and to validate treatment efficacy. Therefore, treatment-outcome monitoring has gained new importance in health care. Health care professionals are now themselves being monitored to determine the effectiveness of the treatments they provide and evaluate patient satisfaction with their treatment. Often, a scorecard is maintained by third-party payers to monitor practitioners' efficacy (Gatchel & Oordt, 2003). Health care professionals also need to monitor such outcomes for quality-assurance purposes. Data are also needed that can provide third-party payers with demonstrations of treatment efficacy. This can be an important marketing strategy to highlight the effectiveness of one's pain management program.

Unfortunately, many health care professionals do not have a background in conducting program or treatment evaluations because of the requisite experimental methodology and statistical tools needed for such evaluations. One needs to set up a database with appropriate psychometrically sound measures to use at baseline and follow-up evaluations. Such data then need to be statistically analyzed. Fortunately, there are now templates for conducting such evaluations. Gatchel (2001) and Mayer, Prescott, and Gatchel (2000) have provided such overviews. Morley and Williams (2002) also presented a comprehensive review of how to conduct and evaluate treatment outcome studies.

It should also be noted that earlier, Blanchard (1979) highlighted six important dimensions that one should consider in evaluating clinical applications and effectiveness of therapeutic modalities, using biofeedback as an example. These same six dimensions would similarly be appropriate for the evaluation of various pain management procedures. These dimensions consist of the following:

1. The percentage or fraction of the treated patient sample that demonstrated significant therapeutic improvement.
2. The degree of clinical meaningfulness of the therapeutic changes that were obtained.
3. The degree of transfer of changes that were obtained in the clinical setting to the patient's natural environment.
4. The degree of change in the biopsychosocial response for which the treatment was prescribed.
5. The degree of replicability of the results by different clinicians and clinical sites.
6. The extent and thoroughness of the follow-up data for pain.

Each of these dimensions is important and should be considered when evaluating the therapeutic effectiveness of any pain management intervention. Finally, in any discussion of treatment outcomes monitoring, clinicians now need to be aware of the Health Insurance Portability and Accountability Act (HIPAA) privacy rules, reviewed in chapter 10. These rules establish patients' rights concerning the use and disclosure of their health care information (including when it is being used for research outcomes purposes). In addition to the usual informed consent obtained according to each institution's review board monitoring the safety of subjects involved in any clinical research trial, an additional HIPAA consent form must also be obtained. An example of such a form is presented in Appendix 11.2. Health care professionals may order HIPAA privacy rules information and forms from their specialty organizations. For example, HIPAA for Psychologists can be ordered at the Web site http://www.apapractice.org.

COST EFFECTIVENESS OF PAIN MANAGEMENT

Intimately related to the above reviewed topic of treatment outcomes evaluation is the issue of cost effectiveness. For example, chronic pain alone is a very expensive health care item, with estimates as high as $125 million annually for health care and indemnity costs. Specialized pain management programs are usually expensive, averaging $8,100 for comprehensive treatment programs (Marketdata Enterprises, 1995). Thus, if interdisciplinary pain programs are to survive in today's managed-care environment they will need to demonstrate that they are both clinically effective as well as cost effective. Fortunately, there have been systematic evaluations of outcomes related to the issue of cost effectiveness of interdisciplinary pain management programs. For example, Turk and Okifuji (1998) reported on the cost effectiveness of such programs by calculating differences in pain medication, health care utilization, and disability payments. They then compared the outcome of these financial parameters to the most frequently used treatment modalities. Overall, their results demonstrated that pain rehabilitation programs were up to 21 times more cost effective than alternative treatments, such as surgery. Other publications have also reported such savings (see Turk, 2002). It is very worthwhile to provide such scientific data to third-party payers to justify the clinical and cost effectiveness of comprehensive pain management programs.

One should also keep in mind that many treatments for pain involve a wide variety of components delivered in potentially different modalities (e.g., individual vs. group, inpatient vs. outpatient, daily vs. weekly) and may also include different health care providers. To date, very little research has isolated what features are vitally necessary and sufficient to produce the optimal outcomes. Apparently, third-party payers are insisting that health care providers consider cost effectiveness. The trend for evidence-based medicine requires that health care professionals begin to demonstrate the clinical and cost effectiveness of the treatments that are provided (Turk & Gatchel, 1999a). In the future, they need to pay better attention to the issue of both what is necessary and also sufficient to produce the best outcomes with specific pain syndromes. As Gatchel and Herring (2002) noted, the reasons for monitoring evidence-based outcomes include the following:

- To provide objective data to third-party payers to document treatment effectiveness. These data can also be used to market the clinical effectiveness of a practice. For example, there is now evidence for safety, efficacy, and cost effectiveness of evidence-based guidelines for the management of acute low back pain in primary care.

- To monitor the quality assurance in one's own practice. Regular evaluation of treatment outcomes allows the practitioners to ascertain whether there is any slippage in the quality of care being provided.
- For those interested in contributing to the scientific literature, such evidence-based outcomes serve as a foundation for publication or presentation of data at professional meetings.

DEVELOPMENT OF EARLY PREVENTION AND INTERVENTION STRATEGIES TO PREVENT CHRONIC PAIN PROBLEMS

Linton (2002) discussed the great advantages of early prevention and intervention for acute pain to prevent the development of chronic pain disability problems. Indeed, there have been a number of preliminary studies suggesting the success of such an approach. However, as Linton and Bradley (1996) pointed out, although cost reduction is often used as an argument for early intervention programs, there has been a paucity of adequate analyses reported in the literature. For example, Goossens and Evers (1997) noted this paucity in the area of low back pain. The few analyses that have been reported, though, have suggested such savings (cited in Linton & Bradley, 1996). For instance, Mitchell and Carmen (1990) presented preliminary findings from a multicenter trial (involving more than 3,000 patients with acute soft tissue and back injuries). Two groups of patients were compared: (a) those who received early intensive intervention and (b) those who received standard treatments at other facilities. During a 5-month follow-up period, it was found that there was a savings *each* month of roughly $1 million to $1.5 million in wage loss and health care costs. In a follow-up evaluation of 542 patients, Mitchell and Carmen (1994) found that the early intensive intervention produced a projected savings of $5,000/patient. As Linton and Bradley (1996) concluded in their review of the literature, these early data suggest that it is indeed possible to prevent the development of chronic disability:

> However, if this goal is to be met, we need to continue to make bold attempts—both clinically and scientifically—to provide effective secondary prevention measures. Research to date has provided a very good beginning, but details have yet to be worked out. If the promise of prevention is to be fully realized, these details are urgently needed. (p. 454)

In a study that has made a significant stride in this area, my colleagues and I (Gatchel et al., 2003) reported that early intervention at the acute stage of low back pain significantly reduced the prevalence of future chronic disability problems, relative to acute low back pain patients who did not receive any such early intervention. We found that high-risk acute low back pain patients who received early intervention displayed significantly fewer indications of chronic pain disability at a 1-year follow-up on a wide range of work, health care utilization, medication use, and self-reported pain variables, relative to high-risk acute low back pain patients who did not receive such early intervention. For example, we found that the early intervention group was much more likely to have returned to work (at about a 4.5 times greater rate) and was also about one half times less likely to be taking narcotic analgesics, relative to individuals who did not receive early intervention. Moreover, there was a significant cost savings of the early intervention program. At the 1-year follow-up, the average cost of treatment and work disability days/lost wages was approximately $12,000 for the early intervention group, as contrasted to approximately $22,000 for the non-early intervention group patients. These results have obvious major implications in terms of decreasing the emotional distress and producing socioeconomic cost savings for this prevalent pain disability problem. More research of this type, with other types of pain syndromes, is needed because of the potential savings in cost as well as in emotional distress of patients.

COMORBID PAIN AND MENTAL HEALTH PROBLEMS

Well-documented clinical evaluations have concluded that patients with chronic pain also manifest concurrent psychiatric illness, most commonly depression, anxiety disorders, and substance abuse disorders (Dersh, Polatin, & Gatchel, 2002). Also, there are close associations among chronic pain, depression, and suicide. Patients with chronic pain are at increased risk for depression (Rush, Polatin, & Gatchel, 2000); suicide (Fishbain, 1999; Parker, 1998), which has been identified by the U.S. Surgeon General as one of the top public health concerns in the country; and sleep disorders (Hanscom & Jex, 2001). As pain becomes more chronic, emotional factors play an increasingly dominant role in the maintenance of dysfunction and suffering (Dersh et al., 2002). More work is needed that focuses on the most effective means of dealing with this comorbidity.

All pain management approaches, therefore, require a strong mental health component, which can be directed by a psychiatrist or clinical psychologist. Indeed, the most efficacious interdisciplinary intervention approaches involve cognitive–behavioral treatment components. This further attests to the major role that mental health issues play in pain management. Moreover, this strong emphasis on mental health is also evidenced by the potentially common pathogenetic mechanisms involved in some psychiatric disorders, such as depression and pain. For example, the physiological similarities between chronic pain and depression have been well documented. Both nociceptive and affective pathways coincide anatomically in these syndromes. Furthermore, norepinephrine and serotonin, the two neurotransmitters most often implicated in the pathophysiology of mood disorders, are also involved in the gate-control mechanisms of pain. Antidepressants have also been found to be effective in the treatment of some chronic-pain patients.

It should also be noted that there is currently a need for a strong mental health life span emphasis at this time. Chronic physical and mental health problems have become significant for elderly individuals and, as mentioned earlier, the prevalence of such conditions can be expected to increase as the U.S. population ages. Epidemiologic projections suggest a chronic-pain prevalence of at least 2% of the adult population (Verhaak, Kerssens, Dekker, Sorbi, & Bensing, 1998). Awareness of these population trends is contributing to an increased concern about health care for older adults, which will include mental health and pain problems.

COMPLEMENTARY AND ALTERNATIVE MEDICINE APPROACHES TO PAIN MANAGEMENT

The general population is beginning to more widely utilize various alternative or complementary medicine approaches. These approaches can be defined as medical interventions that are not usually taught widely in U.S. medical schools and that are not generally available in hospitals. Examples of such approaches include acupuncture, massage, and chiropractic and various herbal remedies. In point of fact, many herbal remedies (see Figure 11.1) have been used for centuries in Europe (Sanides, 2003). In a very influential survey on the use of such approaches in the United States, Eisenberg et al. (1993) reported that an estimated 60 million Americans used such alternative medical therapies in 1990, at an estimated cost of $13.7 billion. In addition, the estimated number of annual visits to providers of alternative medicine amounted to 425 million visits, which far exceeded the number of visits to all primary-care physicians in the United States (388 million visits). Another important finding is that 70% of patients who acknowledged using alternative therapy never mentioned it to their physicians. These data stimulated a great deal of attention and debate regarding this "invisible mainstream" that exists within the U.S. health care system.

Many misconceptions remain about alternative or complementary medicine. In the past, it has often been viewed as some sort of "fringe" medicine. However, this is far from the truth. Alternative or complementary

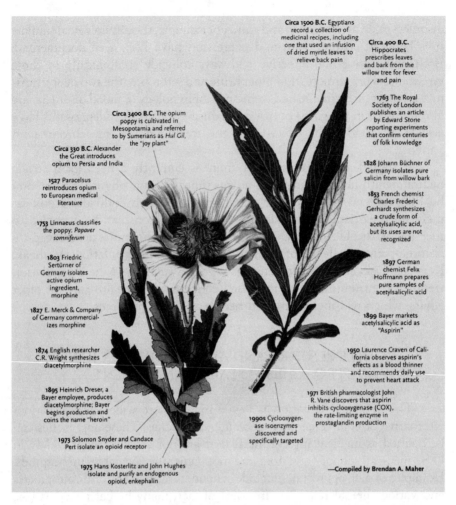

Circa 1500 B.C. Egyptians record a collection of medicinal recipes, including one that used an infusion of dried myrtle leaves to relieve back pain

Circa 400 B.C. Hippocrates prescribes leaves and bark from the willow tree for fever and pain

1763 The Royal Society of London publishes an article by Edward Stone reporting experiments that confirm centuries of folk knowledge

Circa 3400 B.C. The opium poppy is cultivated in Mesopotamia and referred to by Sumerians as *Hul Gil*, the "joy plant"

Circa 330 B.C. Alexander the Great introduces opium to Persia and India

1527 Paracelsus reintroduces opium to European medical literature

1753 Linnaeus classifies the poppy: *Papaver somniferum*

1803 Friedric Sertürner of Germany isolates active opium ingredient, morphine

1827 E. Merck & Company of Germany commercializes morphine

1874 English researcher C.R. Wright synthesizes diacetylmorphine

1895 Heinrich Dreser, a Bayer employee, produces diacetylmorphine; Bayer begins production and coins the name "heroin"

1973 Solomon Snyder and Candace Pert isolate an opioid receptor

1975 Hans Kosterlitz and John Hughes isolate and purify an endogenous opioid, enkephalin

1828 Johann Büchner of Germany isolates pure salicin from willow bark

1853 French chemist Charles Frederic Gerhardt synthesizes a crude form of acetylsalicylic acid, but its uses are not recognized

1897 German chemist Felix Hoffmann prepares pure samples of acetylsalicylic acid

1899 Bayer markets acetylsalicylic acid as "Aspirin"

1950 Laurence Craven of California observes aspirin's effects as a blood thinner and recommends daily use to prevent heart attack

1971 British pharmacologist John R. Vane discovers that aspirin inhibits cyclooxygenase (COX), the rate-limiting enzyme in prostaglandin production

1990s Cyclooxygenase isoenzymes discovered and specifically targeted

—Compiled by Brendan A. Maher

Figure 11.1. Plants for pain. From "Plants for Pain," by B. A. Maher, 2003, *The Scientist, 17*(25), p. 25. Copyright 2003 by The Scientist LLL. Reprinted with permission.

medicine is an important area within medicine. It is merely a continuation of the tradition of medicine that incorporates new approaches that have been demonstrated on the basis of scientific research to be efficacious. For example, therapies based on herbs have been used to treat various medical problems for hundreds of years. The Chinese practice of acupuncture also has a long history. In fact, the National Institutes of Health now has an Office of Complementary and Alternative Medicine, which focuses on helping to stimulate new research in this area of medicine. Conventional medicine has been historically slow to embrace new concepts and treatment approaches. Alternative or complementary medicine is an example of a new area that is slowly being embraced. Indeed, a national trend has developed in which some third-party payers authorize alternative therapies in the form of expanded benefits (Eisenberg, 1997).

As noted earlier, one of the striking findings of Eisenberg et al.'s (1993) study was the fact that 70% of patients who were using alternative or complementary therapies never mentioned it to their physicians. This has created a potential health care problem because, for example, certain over-the-counter herbal remedies can duplicate medically prescribed drugs. As a case in point, St. John's Wort is publicized as having a beneficial effect in reducing depression. If a patient is taking St. John's Wort (and does not tell his or her physician about it), and then is prescribed an antidepressant for symptoms of depression and sleeplessness, the patient will be getting a double dose of a drug that can result in potentially toxic levels (Eisenberg, 1997). Physicians therefore need to evaluate patients fully for their possible use of alternative medical therapies. Eisenberg (1997) provided a comprehensive step-by-step strategy for conventionally trained medical providers to use with their patients to proactively discuss the use or avoidance of alternative therapies. This strategy involves the following:

- Review safety and efficacy issues related to alternative medical therapies. For example, the potential toxicity of herbal preparations, dietary regimens and supplements, and so on, is important to review with patients. Request that patients maintain a symptom diary if they are using alternative medical therapies, which can be used to conduct a baseline assessment and follow-up evaluation of a subsequent alternative or conventional therapeutic intervention.
- For patients who are using alternative medical therapies, arrange for follow-up visits to monitor for potentially harmful side effects.

The U.S. population includes a large number of users of alternative medical therapies. In the past, such therapies have been ignored by physicians of conventional medicine. They can no longer be ignored. Therefore, careful monitoring of the use of such therapies is essential so that some of the conventional medical procedures that may be prescribed will not be negatively affected. Obviously, this type of monitoring will require some additional evaluation and discussion between patients and health care professionals.

A number of alternative medicine approaches are beginning to be used for the treatment of pain. Berman, Jonas, and Swyers (1998) reviewed research on the efficacy of alternative medicine therapies such as acupuncture and chiropractic and various mind–body techniques for treating various chronic pain syndromes. One of the traditional approaches has been biofeedback. Keep in mind, though, that many times these approaches cannot be used as the sole treatment modality. Rather, they should be used as complementary approaches with other conventional approaches. Other alternative or complementary approaches that are beginning to be used in the area of pain management include hypnosis, massage therapy, and herbalism. Also, recent studies have demonstrated the effectiveness of acupuncture for low back pain. In one such study, Ghoname et al. (1999) compared the effectiveness of percutaneous electrical nerve stimulation (PENS), which is a form of acupuncture, to transcutaneous electrical nerve stimulation and low back exercise therapies in patients with chronic low back pain. A sham PENS procedure was also included in the design to control for possible placebo effects. A pre- to posttreatment assessment randomized design was used. The results clearly demonstrated that the acupuncture (PENS) treatment was significantly more effective in decreasing self-reported pain and medication use as well as in improving physical activity, quality of sleep, and a sense of well-being, relative to the other three conditions. Moreover, 81% of the patients stated that they would be willing to pay money out of pocket to receive PENS therapy, compared to only 4% to 9% who stated this regarding the other treatment modalities.

For readers who are interested in further reviews of alternative or complementary medicine, there is a growing list of publications available. In the area of pain treatment, Davis (1997) presented a number of alternative/complementary modalities that can be used by physical therapists and other health care professionals in the management of chronic pain patients. More recently, Berman (2004) edited a Special Topic Series on the use of complementary and alternative approaches to pain.

MOTIVATION FOR, AND COMPLIANCE WITH, PAIN MANAGEMENT PROGRAMS

In chapter 7, I discussed the important role of motivation in pain management. As Turk and Gatchel (1999b) highlighted, there is still a great need for research focusing on the role of psychosocial, affective, cognitive, and behavioral factors in the initial acceptance of a treatment program, and motivation for self-management techniques often required in such programs, as well as adherence to such programs. More specific assessment methods need to be developed to identify individual impediments to treatment responsiveness and patients' receptiveness to programs. Techniques to prevent relapse are also important. Relapse-prevention models, such as those originally developed by Marlatt and Gordon (1980, 1985), are greatly needed to address the problem of long-term maintenance of the gains in new health behaviors introduced in pain management programs. Of course, closely aligned with the issue of relapse prevention is the important issue of adherence. A clinician may have the best treatment program in the world, but if he or she fails to be certain that patients will adhere to such a program, then he or she cannot expect success. Health care professionals need to attend to the individual characteristics of their patients, focusing on those who will adhere versus those who will not, in order to tailor their program to capture all of their patients.

PAIN MANAGEMENT STANDARDS

In 2002, the American Pain Society deemed it essential that a high priority was to develop evidence-based and cost-effective goals to improve the quality of pain management (Miaskowski, 2002). This would then, it is hoped, lead to the establishment of a clinical practice guideline program that would serve as a template for the consistent application of the most proven and up-to-date assessment and treatment techniques. This is greatly needed in today's environment, in which third-party payers are attempting to reduce health care costs at the expense of patients and professionals. Health care professionals need to present a united front in putting their best foot forward in attacking these short-sighted penny-wise but dollar-foolish approaches that are leading to more long-term chronic problems by focusing on only the most inexpensive. short-term fixes. Indeed, as I discussed in chapter 10, reimbursement issues are becoming a major survival concern for pain management professionals. Only if pain management professionals approach this threat as a united front, with the best evidence-based pain management techniques available, will they have a chance to compete in the marketplace. As Loeser (2001) appropriately noted, the future survival of pain management as a specialty will depend on the following:

- Pain management professionals must develop effective clinical guidelines based on solid outcomes research.
- In today's climate of cost containment, they must demonstrate the cost effectiveness of their services.
- They must demonstrate to the public that they provide effective pain management services.
- They must lobby the government and fight for appropriate funding for their services.

SUMMARY

The development of both treatment- and cost-effective pain management programs has come a long way during the past decade. On the basis

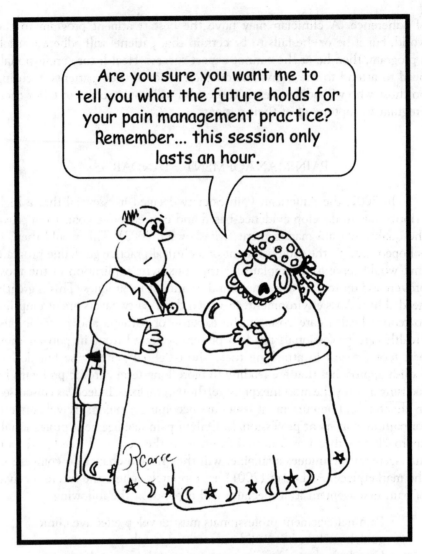

There are many issues and topics that require additional attention in the future because of their important clinical relevance.

of the biopsychosocial model, it is now evident that pain is a complex problem requiring consideration of potentially complex interactions between biological and psychosocial variables. When these pain syndromes become chronic in nature, they often cannot be cured, but merely treated or managed. To prevent such chronic conditions from developing, care must be taken to provide a more active preventive approach and to be more proactive in dealing with the acute pain problem before it spirals into a more complex, chronic biopsychosocial problem. The pain management community of professionals is now poised to embrace this biopsychosocial perspective and integrate it into their practices. An important arena for future advances is in the primary-care setting; this is where cost containment can be initiated by preventing the development of chronic pain problems. Close collaboration between primary-care physicians and pain management specialists will likely go a long way in the early identification and prevention of patients with pain who are at high risk for developing more chronic pain disability problems. Continued clinical research in this area will, it is hoped, lead to even a better understanding of pain in order to prevent disability as well as to treat the diverse conditions that come under the generic rubric of pain. This evolution will require consistent efforts by pain management specialists to better understand the etiology, assessment, and treatment of all types of pain at the acute, subacute, and chronic levels of development. Moreover, the development and consistent use of a standard clinical practice guideline program, based on evidence-based outcomes, is greatly needed for the economic survival of pain management specialists.

REFERENCES

Berman, B. (2004). Special topics series. *Complementary and Alternative Medicine*, 20, 1–32.

Berman, B. M., Jonas, W., & Swyers, J. P. (1998). Issues in the use of complementary/alternative medical therapies for low back pain. *Physical Medicine & Rehabilitation Clinics of North America, 9*, 497–513.

Blanchard, E. B. (1979). Biofeedback and the modification of cardiovascular dysfunctions. In R. J. Gatchel & K. P. Price (Eds.), *Clinical applications of biofeedback: Appraisal and status* (pp. 28–51). New York: Pergamon Press.

Davis, C. M. (Ed.). (1997). *Complementary therapies and rehabilitation.* Thorofare, NJ: Slack.

Dersh, J., Polatin, P., & Gatchel, R. (2002). Chronic pain and psychopathology: Research findings and theoretical considerations. *Psychosomatic Medicine, 64*, 773–786.

Eisenberg, D. M. (1997). Advising patients who seek alternative medical therapies [see comments]. *Annals of Internal Medicine, 127*, 61–69.

Eisenberg, D. M., Kessler, R. C., Foster, C., Norlock, F. E., Calkins, D. R., & Delbanco, T. L. (1993). Unconventional medicine in the United States. *New England Journal of Medicine, 328*, 246–252.

Epker, J., & Gatchel, R. J. (2000). Coping profile differences in the biopsychosocial functioning of TMD patients. *Psychosomatic Medicine, 62*, 69–75.

Etscheidt, M. A., Steiger, H. G., & Braverman, B. (1995). Multidimensional Pain Inventory profile classifications and psychopathology. *Journal of Consulting and Clinical Psychology, 51*, 29–36.

Fishbain, D. (1999). The association of chronic pain and suicide. *Seminars in Clinical Neuropsychiatry, 4,* 221–227.

Gatchel, R. J. (1999). Perspectives on pain: A historical overview. In R. J. Gatchel & D. C. Turk (Eds.), *Psychosocial factors in pain: Critical perspectives* (pp. 3–17). New York: Guilford Press.

Gatchel, R. J. (2001). A biopsychosocial overview of pre-treatment screening of patients with pain. *Clinical Journal of Pain, 17,* 192–199.

Gatchel, R. J., & Herring, S. A. (2002). Evidenced-based medicine. In A. J. Cole & S. A. Herring (Eds.), *The low back pain handbook* (2nd ed., pp. 533–538). Philadelphia: Hanley & Belfus.

Gatchel, R. J., & Oordt, M. S. (2003). *Clinical health psychology and primary care: Practical advice and clinical guidance for successful collaboration.* Washington, DC: American Psychological Association.

Gatchel, R. J., Polatin, P. B., Noe, C. E., Gardea, M. A., Pulliam, C., & Thompson, J. (2003). Treatment- and cost-effectiveness of early intervention for acute low back pain patients: A one-year prospective study. *Journal of Occupational Rehabilitation, 13,* 1–9.

Ghoname, E. A., Craig, W. F., White, P. F., Ahmed, H. E., Hamza, M. A., Henderson, B. N., et al. (1999). Percutaneous electrical nerve stimulation for low back pain: A randomized crossover study. *Journal of the American Medical Association, 281,* 818–823. [Published erratum appears in *Journal of the American Medical Association,* 1999, *281,* p. 1795]

Goossens, M. E. J. B., & Evers, S. M. A. A. (1997). Economic evaluation of back pain interventions. *Journal of Occupational Rehabilitation, 7,* 15–32.

Hanscom, D., & Jex, R. (2001). Sleep disorders, depression and musculoskeletal pain. *Spineline, 2*(5), 56–59.

Kerns, R. D., Rosenberg, R., Jamison, R. N., Caudill, M. A., & Haythornthwaite, J. A. (1997). Readiness to adopt a self-management approach to chronic pain: The Pain Stages of Change Questionnaire (PSOCQ). *Pain, 72,* 227–234.

Kerns, R. D., Turk, D. C., & Rudy, T. E. (1985). The West Haven–Yale Multidimensional Pain Inventory. *Pain, 23,* 345–356.

Linton, S. J. (2002). A cognitive–behavioral approach to the prevention of chronic back pain. In D. C. Turk & R. J. Gatchel (Eds.), *Psychological approaches to pain management: A practitioner's handbook* (2nd ed., pp. 317–333). New York: Guilford Press.

Linton, S. J., & Bradley, L. A. (1996). Strategies for the prevention of chronic pain. In R. J. Gatchel & D. C. Turk (Eds.), *Psychological approaches to pain management: A practitioner's handbook* (pp. 438–457). New York: Guilford Press.

Loeser, J. D. (2001). The future: Will pain be abolished or just pain specialists? *APA Bulletin, 11,* 1–10.

Marketdata Enterprises. (1995). *Chronic pain management programs: A market analysis.* Valley Stream, NY: Author.

Marlatt, G. A., & Gordon, J. R. (1980). Determinants of relapse: Implications for the maintenance of behavior change. In P. O. Davidson & S. M. Davidson (Eds.), *Behavioral medicine: Changing health lifestyles* (pp. 145–161). New York: Brunner/Mazel.

Marlatt, G. A., & Gordon, J. R. (Eds.). (1985). *Relapse prevention: Maintenance strategies in the treatment of addictive behaviors.* New York: Guilford Press.

Mayer, T. G., Gatchel, R. J., & Polatin, P. B. (Eds.). (2000). *Occupational musculoskeletal disorders: Function, outcomes and evidence.* Philadelphia: Lippincott, Williams & Wilkins.

Mayer, T. G., Prescott, M., & Gatchel, R. J. (2000). Objective outcomes evaluation: Methods and evidence. In T. G. Mayer, P. B. Polatin, & R. J. Gatchel (Eds.), *Occupational musculoskeletal disorders: Function, outcomes, and evidence* (pp. 651–667). Philadelphia: Lippincott, Williams & Wilkins.

Miaskowski, C. (2002). President's message: APS board of directors revises strategic plan. *APS Bulletin, 12,* 2–4.

Mitchell, R. I., & Carmen, G. M. (1990). Results of a multicenter trial using an intensive active exercise program for the treatment of acute soft tissue and back injuries. *Spine, 15,* 514–521.

Mitchell, R. I., & Carmen, G. M. (1994). The functional restoration approach to the treatment of chronic pain in patients with soft tissue and back injuries. *Spine, 19,* 633–642.

Morley, S., & Williams, A. D. C. (2002). Conducting and evaluating treatment outcome studies. In D. C. Turk & R. J. Gatchel (Eds.), *Psychological approaches to pain management: A practitioner's handbook* (2nd ed., pp. 52–68). New York: Guilford Press.

Parker, S. (1998, October 21). Seeing suicide as preventable: A national strategy emerges. *Christian Science Monitor,* 3.

Prochaska, J. O., & DiClemente, C. C. (1983). Stages and processes of self-change in smoking: Toward an integrative model. *Journal of Consulting and Clinical Psychology, 51,* 390–395.

Rush, A., Polatin, P., & Gatchel, R. J. (2000). Depression and chronic low back pain: Establishing priorities in treatment. *Spine, 25,* 2566–2571.

Sanides, S. (2003, June 2). A peek inside a medieval medicine cabinet. *The Scientist,* 9.

Turk, D. C. (1990). Customizing treatment for chronic pain patients: Who, what, and why. *Clinical Journal of Pain, 6,* 225–270.

Turk, D. C. (2002). Clinical effectiveness and cost effectiveness of treatment for patients with chronic pain. *Clinical Journal of Pain, 18,* 355–365.

Turk, D. C., & Gatchel, R. J. (1999a). Multidisciplinary programs for rehabilitation of chronic low back pain patients. In W. H. Kirkaldy-Willis & T. N. Bernard Jr. (Eds.), *Managing low back pain* (4th ed., pp. 299–311). New York: Churchill Livingstone.

Turk, D. C., & Gatchel, R. J. (1999b). Psychosocial factors and pain: Revolution and evolution. In R. J. Gatchel & D. C. Turk (Eds.), *Psychosocial factors in pain: Critical perspectives* (pp. 481–493). New York: Guilford Press.

Turk, D. C., & Monarch, E. S. (2002). Biopsychosocial perspective on chronic pain. In D. C. Turk & R. J. Gatchel (Eds.), *Psychological approaches to pain management: A practitioner's handbook* (2nd ed., pp. 3–29). New York: Guilford Press.

Turk, D. C., & Okifuji, A. (1998). Treatment of chronic pain patients: Clinical outcomes, cost-effectiveness, and cost–benefits of multidisciplinary pain centers. *Critical Reviews in Physical and Rehabilitation Medicine, 10,* 181–208.

Turk, D. C., & Okifuji, A. (2001). Matching treatment to assessment of patients with chronic pain. In D. C. Turk & R. Melzack (Eds.), *Handbook of pain assessment* (2nd ed., pp. 400–414). New York: Guilford Press.

Turk, D. C., Okifuji, A., Sinclair, J. D., & Starz, T. W. (1998). Interdisciplinary treatment for fibromyalgia syndrome: Clinical and statistical significance. *Arthritis Care & Research, 11,* 186–195.

U.S. Census Bureau. (2000). *Population projections of the United States by age, sex, race, Hispanic origin, and nativity: 1999 to 2100.* Washington, DC: Author.

U.S. Census Bureau. (2001). *The 65 years and over population: 2000.* Washington, DC: Author.

Verhaak, P. F. M., Kerssens, J. J., Dekker, J., Sorbi, M. J., & Bensing, J. M. (1998). Prevalence of chronic benign pain disorder among adults: A review of the literature. *Pain, 77,* 231–239.

APPENDIX 11.1

Recommended Readings

Dersh, J., Polatin, P., & Gatchel, R. (2002). Chronic pain and psychopathology: Research findings and theoretical considerations. *Psychosomatic Medicine*, 64, 773–786.

Eisenberg, D. M. (1997). Advising patients who seek alternative medical therapies [see comments]. *Annals of Internal Medicine*, 127, 61–69.

Gatchel, R. J., Polatin, P. B., Noe, C. E., Gardea, M. A., Pulliam, C., & Thompson, J. (2003). Treatment- and cost-effectiveness of early intervention for acute low back pain patients: A one-year prospective study. *Journal of Occupational Rehabilitation*, 13, 1–9.

Linton, S. J., & Bradley, L. A. (1996). Strategies for the prevention of chronic pain. In R. J. Gatchel & D. C. Turk (Eds.), *Psychological approaches to pain management: A practitioner's handbook* (pp. 438–457). New York: Guilford Press.

Loeser, J. D. (2001). The future: Will pain be abolished or just pain specialists? *APA Bulletin*, 11, 1–10.

Morley, S., & Williams, A. D. C. (2002). Conducting and evaluating treatment outcome studies. In D. C. Turk & R. J. Gatchel (Eds.), *Psychological approaches to pain management: A practitioner's handbook* (2nd ed., pp. 53–68). New York: Guilford Press.

APPENDIX 11.2

HIPAA Consent Form for Use of Client Health Information in Clinical Research and Monitoring

PUT NAME OF INSTITUTION HERE

Authorization for Use and Disclosure of Protected Health Information for Research Purposes

1. You agree to permit *[Institution/Covered Entity]* to release your protected health information to *[Name of Principal Investigator]* and his/her staff ("Researchers") for the purpose of conducting the medical research study ***[Abbreviated** title*, IRB #, plus **Brief** *description—e.g., comparative study of two treatments for recurrent breast cancer.]*

2. You agree to permit *[Name of Principal Investigator]* and his/her staff to receive health information about you, and to use and disclose that information to the sponsor of the research, *[Name of Sponsor]*, and representatives of the sponsor, *[Name(s) of Organization(s)—e.g., Contract Research Organization(s), Reference Laboratory(-ies)]*, assisting in the research ("Receiver[s]").

3. When we talk about protected health information about you to be used and disclosed, it includes all information about you collected during the research study for research purposes and the protected health information about you in medical records that is related to the research study. *[List types of medical information that will be collected, used, and disclosed—e.g., blood, urine, and bone marrow tests, x-ray examinations, etc.]*

4. Protected health information about you may also be disclosed to and reviewed by a research ethics board and representatives of government agencies, including the Food and Drug Administration (FDA) and the Office of Human Research Protections (OHRP) in order to ensure that the research is being conducted in accord with legal and ethical standards. If protected health information about you is required, the reviewers may need your entire medical record.

5. Protected health information about you may also be used to create information that does not identify you. The de-identified data may be used and released by Researchers, including use for other research purposes.

6. You understand that your protected health information may be further disclosed to someone who is not required to comply with the federal privacy protection regulations. If so, the state and federal privacy regulations may no longer protect your information and it may be subject to re-disclosure.

7. In order to participate in this research study, you must sign this Authorization. However, you cannot be denied medical treatment, payment of, or eligibility for, benefits because you did not sign this Authorization.

8. This Authorization has no expiration date.

9. You have the right to revoke this Authorization at any time by a written notification to: *[Principal Investigator or Designee, address, and phone number]*

10. A copy of this authorization form will be provided to you.

If you revoke this Authorization, you will no longer be allowed to participate in the research. Also, even if you revoke this Authorization, the Researchers may still use and disclose the protected health information that they have already obtained as necessary to maintain the reliability of the research.

_____   _____

Signature of Research Participant   Date

_____

Printed Name of Research Participant

For Personal Representative of the Research Participant (if applicable)

Printed Name of Personal Representative: _____

Describe Personal Representative Relationship:

_____

(e.g., parent, guardian, person with power of attorney, etc.)

I certify that I have the legal authority under applicable law to make this Authorization on behalf of the Research Participant identified above.

_____   _____
Signature of Personal Representative   Date

AUTHOR INDEX

Numbers in italics refer to listings in the reference sections.

SUBJECT INDEX

Medication Responsibility Agreement,
199–200, 216–217
Medico–legal jurisdiction, 250–251
Mental filtering, definition, 68, 137
Mental health care reimbursement,
243
Mental health problems, comorbidity,
268–269
Meperidine, 202
Methadone, 202, 204
Migraine headache, management, 57–59
Millon Behavioral Health Inventory, 97–
98, 100–101
Millon Behavioral Medicine Diagnostic,
98
Mind–body relationship, history, 4–7
Mind reading, definition, 68, 71, 137
Mini mental status examination, 94–95,
108–109
Minimal-therapist-contact treatment
headache, 59, 73–76
major components, 73–76
Minimization, definition, 69, 137
Minnesota Multiphasic Personality
Inventory—2, 93–94
Monoamine oxydase inhibitors, 206–207
Morphine, 202–204. See also Opioid medications
Morphine pumps
case vignette, 154–155
in palliative care, 229–230
Motivation, 175–196
clinical interview assessment, 95
intervention strategies, 179–186
secondary gain issues, 121
and self-management of pain,
184–185
stages-of-change model application,
176–177
transtheoretical model, 183
Motivational enhancement therapy,
179–186
caveats, 183–184
phases, 181–183
Motivational interviewing, 178–179
basic principles, 178–179
caveats, 183–184
Motrin, 205
Multidimensional Pain Inventory, 96–97,
100–101, 263
Muscle relaxants, 209–210

Muscle tension, and treatment matching,
39–40

Nalfon, 205
Naproxen (Naprosyn), 205
Narcotics. See Opioid medications
National Health Interview Survey, 3
Neck-and-shoulder pain, case vignette,
147–150
Negative thinking, 130–135
coping thoughts distinction,
133–136
feelings link, 130–133, 138–139
patient/family information, 66–68,
130–136
Nerve blocks, 228
Network event, job loss as, 125
Neuroleptics, 211
Neuromatrix model of pain, 11–13
Neurontin, 210
Neuropathic pain
case vignette, 152–154
management techniques, 38–39
pharmacotherapy, 201, 208
spinal cord stimulation, 228
Nociception
in biopsychosocial model, 13–14
definition, 14, 92
disease analogy, 15
perception of, 92
Nociceptive pain, management, 38
Nonsteroidal anti-inflammatory drugs,
205–206
Numerical rating scales, 54
Nursing services, and treatment team, 61

Occupational therapist, and treatment
team, 61–62
Opioid medications, 202–204, 225–234
addiction issues, 198–200, 218–221,
230–231
biopsychosocial approach, 200–201
cancer pain, 231–234
guidelines, 203–204
history, 270
indications and dosages, 202–203
injection procedures, 225–228
and litigation, 230
in palliative care, 202, 225–234

Physical examination, 33
Physical therapist, and treatment team, 61
Physician and treatment team, 60–61
Physiological pain measures, 27–28
Piroxicam (Feldene), 205
Placebo effect, potential of, 118–119
Plants for pain, 270
Pleasant activity scheduling, 115–117
Polypharmacology
    side effects, 212–213
    use of, 201
Posttraumatic stress symptoms, case
    vignette, 151–152
Preauthorization/precertification nuances,
    247–248
Precontemplation stage of change, 176–
    177, 264
Predictive validity, 29
Preferred-provider networks, 247–248
Prevention strategies, 267–268
Primary care setting
    acute pain management, 55–56
    back pain management shortcom-
        ings, 40–42
    underprescription of opioids, 200
Primary gain, versus secondary gain,
    119–120
Primary intervention, 52–53, 111–112
Primary provider financial model, 242
Privacy protection, 252, 257–258, 265,
    279–281
Prodromal symptoms, headache diaries,
    74
Profiling. See Treatment matching
Progressive muscle relaxation
    general guidelines, 81–83
    headache management, 73–74
Protected health information (PHI),
    257–258
Psychoanalytic theory, of secondary gain,
    119–120
Psychogenic pain, 141
Psychological CPT codes, 243–244
Psychologist, and treatment team, 61
Psychometrics, pain measures, 28–30
Psychopathology, management approach,
    143
Psychotic symptoms, case vignette,
    156–157
Public relations tools, 246–247

"Quick fix" requests, case vignette,
    154–155

Radiographic evaluations, guidelines, 34
Rational polypharmacology, 197
Rational Self-Analysis, 130–133
"Reactivation" treatment, 52, 112
Readiness to change, stage model, 176–
    177, 264
Recurrent pain
    definition, 47–48
    management, 56–59
Reductionism. See Biomedical
    reductionism
Referral sources, 246–247
Refill agreement/policy, 216–218
Reflex sympathetic dystrophy
    case vignette, 151–152
    spinal cord stimulation, 227
Reframing
    in motivational enhancement,
        181–182
    and resistance, 190
Rehabilitation programs, guidelines, 34
Reimbursement/billing issues, 241–258
Relapse prevention, 72–73
    current needs, 272–273
    information for families/patients,
        72–73
    and stages-of-change model, 177
Relaxation training
    headache, 57–58, 73–74
    patient information, 76–86
    protocols, 76–86
    prototypical use of, 115–117
Reliability, pain measures, 28
RESCUE plan, headaches, 75
Resistance
    and motivational interviewing, 179
    strategies for handling, 189–190
Respiratory depression, opioids, 202–203
Resume Worksheet, 170–171
Return-to-work issues, 169
Rheumatological diseases, laboratory test-
    ing, 34–36
Rofecoxib (Vioxx), 205
Roland and Morris Disability Question-
    naire for Low Back Pain, 92,
    100–101
Rolling with resistance, 179, 181–182

definition, 52, 112
in step-care framework, 112–113
Texas Workforce Commission, 169
Thermal biofeedback, headache, 57, 75
Thinking errors, 136–139
Third-party payers, 241–250
    cost–effectiveness evidence for, 266
    reimbursement/billing issues,
        241–250
    treatment outcome monitoring of,
        264
Tolerance to medications, 198
Topical agents, 212
Topiramate (Topamax), 210
Tragabine, 210
Tramadol (Ultram), 202
Transcutaneous electrical nerve stimula-
    tion, 272
Transtheoretical model of change, 183,
    264
Treatment matching
    biopsychosocial approach, 146–147
    current trends, 262–264
    and disease-versus-illness distinction,
        15–16
    personality inventories role, 96–98,
        263
    in psychologically-based pain man-
        agement, 39–40
    and stages-of-change model, 177,
        264
    in step-care framework, 113–115
Treatment outcome, 264–265
    and cost effectiveness demonstra-
        tion, 266–267

important dimensions of, 265
monitoring of, importance, 264–265
and secondary gain, 120–121
Triggerpoint injections, 228
Trileptal, 210
Tylenol 3, 233

Underprescription of opioids, 200, 203,
    230

Validity, pain measures, 28–29
Valproic acid (Depakene), 210
Verbal rating scales, 54
Vioxx, 205
Visual analog scales, 54–55
von Frey's theory, 7–10

West Haven–Yale Multidimensional Pain
    Inventory, 96–97, 100–101
Work transition programs, 147
Workers' compensation
    Medico–legal jurisdictions, 251
    secondary gain issues, 119–122
    state by state variation in evalua-
        tion, 38
Workforce commissions, 169

"You" statements, 71

Zonisamide (Zonegran), 210

ABOUT THE AUTHOR

Robert J. Gatchel, PhD, received his BA in psychology, *summa cum laude,* in 1969, from the State University of New York at Stony Brook, and received his PhD in clinical psychology in 1973 from the University of Wisconsin. He is also a Diplomate of the American Board of Professional Psychology. For the past 20 years, Dr. Gatchel has been the Elizabeth H. Penn Professor of Clinical Psychology and Professor in the Departments of Psychiatry, Anesthesiology and Pain Management, and Rehabilitation Counseling, as well as the Program Director of the Eugene McDermott Center for Pain Management, all at the University of Texas Southwestern Medical Center in Dallas. He is now the chairman of the Department of Psychology at the University of Texas at Arlington. He has conducted extensive evidence-based clinical research, much of it supported by grants from the National Institutes of Health (NIH). He is also the recipient of consecutive Research Scientist Development Awards from NIH. One of his major areas of clinical and research expertise involves the biopsychosocial approach to the etiology, assessment, treatment, and prevention of chronic stress and pain behavior. He has published more than 300 scientific articles and book chapters and has authored or edited 21 books, including *Psychological Approaches to Pain Management: A Practitioner's Handbook, 2nd Edition* (with D. Turk); *Occupational Musculoskeletal Disorders: Function, Outcomes and Evidence* (with T. Mayer & P. Polatin); *The Psychology of Spine Surgery* (with A. Block, W. Deardorff, & R. Guyer); and *Clinical Health Psychology and Primary Care: Practical Advice and Clinical Guidance for Successful Collaboration* (with M. Oordt). Dr. Gatchel is also featured in the *Assessment of Pain*, which is part of the American Psychological Association (APA) Psychotherapy Videotape Series III, "Behavioral Health and Health Counseling" (2002). Finally, Dr. Gatchel has received numerous awards and honors associated with his work in pain assessment and management, including the following: the Volvo Award for Low-Back Pain Research in 1986 from the International Society for the Study of the Lumbar Spine (which is the preeminent international research society for the study of painful spinal disorders); a 1994 Research Award from the North American Spine Society (NASS); the Award for Significant Contributions to Health Psychology, APA Division 38, 1997; NASS's 2001 Henry Farfan Award for Outstanding Contributions to the Field of Spine Care (the first psychologist to receive such an honor); the Award for Outstanding Contributions to the Academy of Behavioral Medicine Research, 2002; and the Award for Significant Contributions to the Field of Temporomandibular Joint and Occlusion Research, 2003. He is also a Visiting Scholar Program awardee, Liberty Mutual Research Center for Safety and Health, Summer 2003, and has received the 2003 Award for Outstanding Contributions to Science from the Texas Psychological Association and the 2004 Award for Distinguished Professional Contributions to Applied Research from APA.